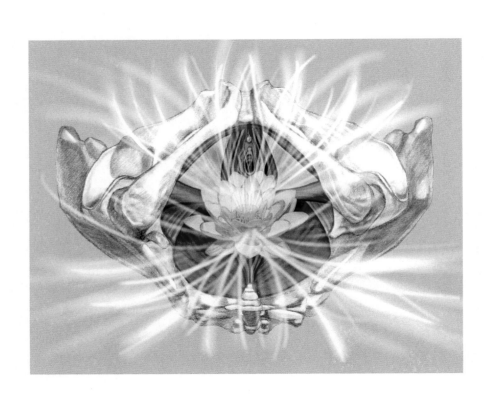

SPIRITUAL ANATOMY

REALIGNING BODY AND SOUL

BY

GINNY NADLER

For my students,
with gratitude—
you birthed and nurtured this modality with me

For Sophie—
you are the future

CONTENTS

INTRODUCTION

BODIES HAVE ALWAYS fascinated me—their structure, their design, what makes them so capable of working well for many years and what makes them decline so dramatically for so many, so quickly. Even as a very young child, I would walk around the apartment spelling b-o-n-e-s incessantly, while my sister screamed, "Mom, make her stop!"

My early fascination with bones and muscles led to the study of anthropology—physical, cultural, and medical. How do the life a person lives and the culture they are born into affect their physical structure? While we all begin with the same basic anatomy, for the most part, the history of our dwelling in our bodies takes different twists and turns and makes us exquisitely unique. I have been called a "body anthropologist," which feels like an apt description for my ongoing quest to understand the sources of our misalignment—both in our own lifetimes and deep in our cultural and evolutionary heritage.

Studying anatomy and dissecting cadavers in school had me in awe. More and more questions constantly emerged as to the mysteries hidden within the body. How movement and the lack of movement actually happen became a deep fascination. Later, I studied embryology and cell biology, and what I discovered felt like a spiritual awakening. The physical body became a window into the spiritual mystery of who we are and where we come from. I have called this book *Spiritual Anatomy* because I see this physical body as the vessel for the Divine energy of consciousness and because, from my perspective, the realignment of the body is what helps to release our spiritual essence to more fully express our soul's destiny in this world.

While I was educating myself in all these ways, my practice of yoga and my studies in the science of yoga were also informing me more deeply about movement patterns. Studying in the school of B.K.S. Iyengar inspired me to sincerely consider this from Mr. Iyengar's teaching: "You must first and foremost see and understand bodies."

Within my yoga classes, I witnessed bodies dramatically out of balance, struggling to "wear" the postures, or asanas, like ill-fitting clothes, on a structure that was distorted and out of alignment. I realized I was doing the same thing myself, and the results were painfully clear in the form of a fast-developing sciatica. Longing to stop fighting my own anatomy, I began an unraveling process that took me deep into the source of our physical misalignment and distortion.

As I released my own body from pain, I started to create a "visual language" to guide students into these areas of physical, emotional, and spiritual congestion. Eventually, I developed my own movement protocol, Structural ReAlignment Integration® (SRI), in order to guide others on this rewarding and healing journey.

The focus of my work is the pelvic floor, and, more specifically, the perineal body within the perineum. I have come to recognize this small, one-inch area as the source of so much distortion, misalignment, and pain. A chronically tight, contracted pelvic floor will congest, spiral, and twist muscle fibers, ultimately pulling the bones out of alignment and leading to pain and dysfunction.

In all the literature and therapies relating to back pain, pelvic floor pain, and other structural pain, I have found few experts who make the connection back to the perineum. Yet as I have guided thousands of people through this protocol in retreats, workshops, and private sessions, I have witnessed again and again the power of beginning with the perineum. You'll meet some of these people in the chapters ahead, and learn about the transformations they experienced as they learned how to create alignment by beginning deep in the pelvic floor.

You may have picked up this book because you yourself are in pain. If so, I hope it will prove to be your doorway to freedom and relief. You may have picked it up because you are a teacher or therapist in a movement modality like yoga, Pilates, or physical therapy. You may have picked it up because you are a medical professional interested in expanding your perceptions of healing. Maybe your calling in life is to help others who are in pain and seeking physical freedom. I hope these pages will be enlightening to you, and I encourage you to include this approach in your specific therapeutic model.

In the chapters that follow, you will learn how our physical distortions are created, why the pelvic floor is so vital, and how you can release the misalignment in your own body. You will be guided to make the important connection between the physical pain you experience and the energetic roadblocks that are deeper in the cell structure, in the very fabric of your being. In Part 1, we will explore the physical, emotional, and spiritual underpinnings of this approach, and in Part 2, I will offer you practical tools to become informed participants in your own "well care," including stretches and guided visualizations. Through practicing these exercises, you will discover how you have created your particular imbalance and learn how to awaken congested places leading to freedom of movement.

Whatever brought you here, it is my intention, as we take this journey together, to guide you to the source of your physical distortion, unraveling the layers to return to your body's natural design. This journey to freedom is not as daunting as it may seem. Once you understand your own anatomy, and how the particular distortions in your body were created through spiraled muscle fibers pulling on your bones, you will breathe a sigh of relief and immediately begin to create space to release stored energy. I hope that as you dance the dance of freedom, joining the moving river of divine energy, you are able to more fully embody your present self and catch glimpses of your future, pain free.

To become the expression of your will, to come home to yourself, is a journey of love. My love for this divine structure we each inhabit has called me to share this possibility for awakening. I am deeply grateful for the opportunity to gift this to you.

ACKNOWLEDGEMENTS

THERE ARE SO many people to whom I want to express my gratitude for their support in the creation of this book. It has been many years in the making. I will attempt to include many from so many chapters of my life, through which I have grown into greater clarity about this precious modality I have been gifted to bring forth. So many have asked me, over twenty-five years or more, "When is the book coming out?" Here it is, my fan club! Thank your all for your ongoing persistence and support. To those that I fail to mention, I am deeply grateful as well—you have all guided me to become an even better bearer of this modality.

Thank you Arlington Smith, my very first collaborator, who felt the potential and possibility of my teaching and created the space for me to birth this pelvic floor modality in New Haven, CT. My students (too many to name) in New Haven who gave life to this work with me in my very first teacher training program, thank you for your faith in me. My students who became collaborators—Tina DiCillo, Anne Ondrey, and Charlotte Wilson in Cleveland, Ohio, and all of the many students who studied with me—I would not have written this book without you. Tom Shaper, who sings my praises at every public event I attend, for example. Ravi Bhandari, you received my wisdom and gifted back to me your committed practice and have been my champion in the writing of this book.

I am grateful to many respected colleagues. Dr. Debra Musso in New York City, as a Network Spinal Doctor, instantly saw the potential for this modality to impact her own work with her practice members. Dr. Tonya Heyman, gynecologist and Women's Health Advocate in Cleveland, Ohio, saw and felt the importance of unraveling the confusion and congestion in the pelvis physically and emotionally. In Texas, Krystyna Jursykowski opened her heart and her doors to bring this work to her community and spread the "word." Philip Beach, osteopath, acupuncturist and embryologist, instantly validated what I viscerally felt to be true about the pelvic floor and the perineum. I am grateful for the opportunity to influence and be influenced by you all.

My thanks also go to my more recent collaborators. Roger Sams, I appreciate your magnificent ability to share with me your expression in dance and provide the space for us to grow our gifts together. Katharine Menton, Goddess of movement awareness in a relational field, thank you for traveling with me and developing our shared expressions more fully to make a greater difference in the lives of others.

To my teachers, who gifted of themselves selflessly, I deeply bow. Dearest Angela Farmer, Goddess Yogini, I awakened to my pelvic floor in your classes over so many years. Ah, those times in Greece. My gratitude goes to you and Victor Van Kooten for coming to my studios to teach over years, and to Kofi Busia for being true to the discipline as our teacher B.K.S. Iyengar intended it to be. And of course, to Mr. Iyengar, who gave so many the gift of discipline. To my very first yoga teacher Larry Hatlett in California who, with his loving peaceful presence and attention to detail, inspired me to teach. To Melinda Perlee, one of my first instructors at the Iyengar Yoga Institute in San Francisco—you probably never knew your effect on my learning. To my teachers at the Iyengar Institute for your guidance, in particular, Judith Lasater, and others over those years. To Felicity Green in Palo Alto, who guided me so well. To Angie Kenny, who knew the indigenous alignment and to Jean Couch who wrote *The Yoga Runner's Book* and understood the importance of the pelvic floor in her teaching. You all influenced me and provided the space for awakening, for me to become the available space for this work to be born and flourish.

My deepest thanks also go to Dr. Bruce Lipton who, through my study of his explorations, paved the way for me to have a clearer understanding of how we came to be who we are. You bridge science and spiritually. To Stephen Busby, who through divine love gifts the WE Space brilliantly for me to expand into even more. To Dr. Keith Jordan, a man who has awakening and higher consciousness as his first priority. Thank you for your leadership, your faith, your sight, and your guidance.

To those who provided friendship and resources over the years to develop Structural ReAlignment Integration—Arlington Smith, Matt and Jean Oristano, Michael and Kareen Caputo, Ann Marie Zaller, and David Klein—thank you for your unwavering belief in my work and in me.

Lisa Chacon, during our first session together, you said "When you write the book..." I responded with "Oh no, not THE BOOK again." You then asked who my editor was and gifted me the introduction to Ellen Daly. Ellen, your commitment to the journey is astounding and your patience with grace incredible! Thank you for riding this whole wave with me and introducing me to Joel Pitney to guide me in the next journey of publication and all that entails. Joel, I am deeply grateful to you for your guidance and for supporting my passion to move into places where this perspective can and will make a difference to many.

I could never have seen into the pelvic floor so clearly without the visionary sight of my artists. Patricia Malcolm, thank you for partnering with me and creating these amazing watercolors of the pelvic anatomy and more. Your illustrations are the living embodiment of the majesty of the pelvis and spine. Thank you also to Susan Viets for stepping into the project when I needed more help. I am deeply grateful. JoAnn Lowe, you received my teachings and became my first artistic collaborator for the DVD "Body So Free" and I have included you here in this book. All of you allow me to see and feel the imbalance on the page that I feel in my body and am expressing in my teachings.

My deepest gratitude goes out to my family. My daughter Jennifer Finkel, who has intimate knowledge of this book writing process, has been my champion and supported me with her deepest love that bridges time. Thank you. My son-in-law Eric Olsen, with Jennifer, provided the space for me to be nourished in family. And Sophie, my granddaughter, provided moments of great relief, reminding me to not take myself so seriously. I deeply love you. My sister Zoe respects me and reminds me of where we came from and all the possibilities to explore.

I am also thankful for my friends Sarah Littlefield and Bruce Abrams, who embraced me into their home and circle, supporting and encouraging me when I arrived in Cleveland. Friendship like ours is not always found. There are so many more friends to honor and the list could go on forever. Robin Cohen, Harriet Slive, Marie and Cliff Hershman, Roseanne and Milton Berkowitz, Sue Livingston, Tina Di Cillo, Anne Ondrey, and Jane Arzt, Bethsaida Ruiz, Katharine Menton, Amy Fox, Adriana Chmiel, Molly Morgan, Pat Malcolm, Susan Viets, Dorothy Tanguay and John McCourt, Frank Setter, thank you all for your deepest love and support and to those of you who provided space for me to write and retreat on occasion. I must single out Forest Jones, Robert Brown, and Meir Schillor—during these years of writing, our weekly calls allow me to soften in your strong presence. I told you on one of those many calls, "You are the best fathers I never had!"

My parents imparted their wisdom in the only way they knew how. I never would have believed that who I have become and the way I see and feel the unfolding of life's mystery is because I am their daughter. They have my eternal gratitude.

I know in the deepest part of me that this creation would never have come into manifestation if it were not for my Spiritual Sangha, creating such a magnificent field for me to be embraced within. Safety has been unearthed for me in community with God and with awakening as my highest priority.

Lastly, my teacher, Thomas Hübl, Modern Mystic, who with the deepest clarity and love has provided the divine field for me to awaken, finding my place of belonging in this divine universe—thank you. I bow down to your divine path and my gratitude is beyond words.

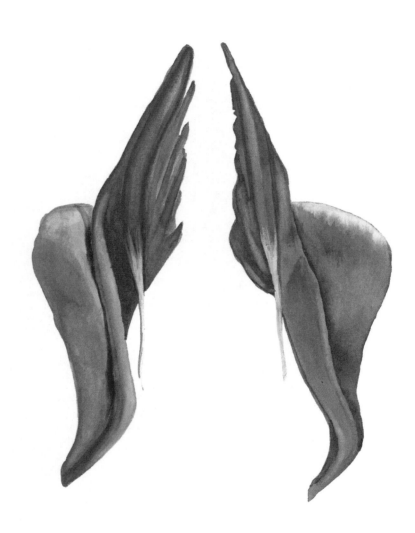

PART I

YOUR BODY TELLS A STORY: UNDERSTANDING HOW YOUR PAIN BEGAN

CHAPTER 1

AN INVITATION TO UNRAVEL

*"We do not heal the past by dwelling there;
we heal the past by living fully in the present."*
—Marianne Williamson

"I DON'T KNOW how you are walking around."

Those were my first words to Judith, an artist in her mid-sixties who came to one of my classes some years ago. It was immediately apparent that simply standing in her body was a great challenge, let alone performing any movement. Her legs were barely able to support her in an upright position. She was bent over and clearly in pain, leaning so far to one side that her balance was very challenged. Indeed, as she told me that day, she had fallen several times, badly. The class began with all of the students lying down on the floor, which was difficult for Judith, however, with support from the other students in the class, she appreciatively surrendered and was able to receive enough instruction to feel where the constriction in the musculature was preventing her from living in free movement. Her pain was profuse, her fear palpable, and yet her desire for change was so great that she had the courage to show up. I must say it was an honor to witness my students holding this dear woman in pure love and possibility.

I suggested she and I work privately. When she walked into my studio that day her demeanor and energy clearly screamed, "Help!" She was depressed, frightened, and appeared to be someone in deep grief.

Everything in Judith's body hurt. She told me that she could no longer pick up her grandchild or move freely in play. And most painful to her was the fact that she was no longer painting. She did not feel the passion nor the ability to express that passion. She felt like she had lost herself. "Where am I? Where did I go?" I could see her desperation to figure out how she got here. How did her body betray her to such a profound extent? How had she ended up in this place of unknowing with no guideposts to direct her back home? Where was the loving, passionate Judith whose very essence sings of joy? She was spiraling down into depression.

"These days that are given to me in life, I cannot do anything with," she told me. "Life is so finite and I am wasting it. Dealing with that thought is shameful. I am here, I am alive, and yet I don't do anything. These days are wasted. My heart cries for the years I have lost."

> *"The future's uncertain and the end is always near."*
> **—Jim Morrison,**
> ***Roadhouse Blues***

My heart ached for Judith. She had been to numerous doctors trying to find the answers to her physical pain. Yet with all the specialists she visited, she didn't feel seen or heard. "I remember them giving far more attention to their computers than to the deplorable state of my health. I have rarely been touched and I feel like most doctors would be happier if I just took antidepressants to feel nothing, to not complain, to not cry out for help."

Judith's pain was physical, but it was also spiritual. She was acutely aware that her very essence was being stifled, and she knew that somehow it was connected to her body—she just did not know how. She intuited that in unlocking her physical contortions she might find her way back to life—back to the dynamic, creative, joyful being that she was, in her essence.

I've met hundreds of people like Judith. Some, like her, have a sense that the ache in their back, the knee pain, the chronic injury is more than just physical. They're ready for a deeper dive into the source of their own pain. Others just want to fix the body and go on their way. All of them, whether they know it or not, are crying out for freedom from a distorted physical structure in which they feel imprisoned.

Let me ask you: Are you in pain? What hurts? Is it a recurring injury, a chronic ache, a growing stiffness? Do you just feel like you can no longer move the way you used to? Are you afraid you're headed for a hip replacement, a cane, or a walker? Do you feel as if your body has betrayed you—like it's no longer a reflection of the person you know you are? Have you accepted your pain, made the best of it, learned to live with it and work around it? Are you traveling to various medical support professionals and other therapists in an attempt to understand your pain? Have you lowered your expectations, told yourself this is just part of getting older? Do you mourn the freedom, ease, and grace you used to feel? Are you frightened?

These are not easy questions to answer, I know. Under the pain lies a fear: What if this is something I have to live with for the rest of my days? What if this limited being is all I am? What if I lose mobility and become dependent on others? What if I can no longer hike, bike, or run, or do any of the other activities I so love? We're afraid to even acknowledge the pain, because then we make ourselves vulnerable to the fear. And fear is just one of the many emotions that we carry in our bodies—along with guilt, shame, and anger.

> *"I am humble enough to say I don't know and committed enough to find out."*
> **—Thomas Hübl**

Judith was lost in a sea of diagnoses, fearful of what she might have to do to regain her self. Mired in the confused structure of her body she felt lost, bereft, and in intense physical agony as she contracted so far away from her divine blueprint. When I looked deeply into Judith's soulful eyes, I could see the joy, the passion, and also the deep sadness blanketing her beautiful light. I knew that our journey together would be one of unraveling the distortions in her physical and emotional body, and giving her deep permission to bring forth that energy and realign anew.

In this book, I hope to guide you on a similar journey. Physical pain is a surface manifestation of much deeper distortions in your body and your being. As such, it is a remarkable opportunity to discover more about your true identity. We live in pain in the outer layers of the musculature, and firmly believe that those aches and intense pains are the cause of the disturbance. It is all we know. Our perception tends to focus on the site of the discomfort; however, where we feel the pain only gives us so much information. This journey will take us through the layers of skin, muscle, fascia, and bone, drawing you deep into the emotional, psychological, cultural, and evolutionary heritage that you carry in every cell of your body. It will not be easy. If you feel trepidation at what you might uncover, that is understandable and appropriate, but the rewards of undertaking this journey are immeasurable. You, in your essence, are a divine being—consciousness embodying itself in a physical form. The goal of our work together will be to liberate that divinity—that energy of awakened consciousness—from the physical blocks that keep it trapped in your body, unable to express itself fully.

I don't know what your potential is when your physical structure comes into profound alignment with the essence of who you are. I don't know my own potential either, but that's what makes this journey so extraordinary. It is open-ended and always humbling in its scope. So let's begin, by reintroducing you to that which is most familiar but in some ways most unknown: your body.

INFORMING THE BODY

Flesh. Organs. Skin. Hair. Bones. And so much more. In my many years studying and working with the human body, I have come to respect its design in ways that I never would have imagined. The body is an extraordinary confluence of life's many dimensions. It is formed of matter, but it is *in*formed by our personal experience, our history, our culture, our environment, and at the deepest level, by divine energy. We are both physical and spiritual beings.

> "We are the swimmers in the divine river, swimming in the sea of creation, and we are what has been created!"
> —**David Abram,**
> *The Spell of the Sensuous*

Imagine that your body is a building. At birth, the spark of divine consciousness that is *you* took up residence in this particular house. We come into this world filled with possibilities and potential, our individual divine blueprint informing us. Over time, however, this "original" movement that guides us so exquisitely is overshadowed by the layers of structure, fear, anger, shame, and shadow that we move through to become embodied.

Each body has a long lineage behind it, not just from our immediate family but from our ancestry. As a global family, humans also carry the legacy of those who preceded us thousands and thousands of years ago. We are each a compilation of many life stories. Our bodies are shaped by our environment—where we happened to land on this earth informs our emotional, physical, and mental composition. Our emotional experiences—traumas and losses as well as the love and nurturing we received—are imprinted on our physicality. The ways we use our bodies also leave their mark. Habitual ways of moving, standing, or sitting; accidents or injuries; sports or other activities—all of these shape the home in which we travel through life. We are like a living encyclopedia, containing all the information from this lifetime and also the entire history of our humanness on this planet and in this universe.

Over the years, our body's natural structure becomes distorted. The body can only support us if there is freedom in the musculature to move around and elongate on the bones. When the muscles become fixed and distorted leading to tension and resistance we are now unable to elongate the bones from behind the musculature into the earth and let the energetic fluid of life's essence flow. We have become locked into the design the fibers have created on the bones. Fluidity is what we all want, to be movers with grace and ease, to be flexible enough that our bones have the space needed to travel through unraveled layers of muscle fiber. Yet, the history that came before us and the years of distortion that we have created most recently have us wearing muscles on bones like clothing that is too tight and is wound in patterns that leave us unable to breathe and be free. Our bones must be free to slide through the muscles like our arms moving through the sleeves of a well-fitting jacket. For most of us, this is not the case.

> *"All memories (wounds and joys) are woven . . . in the human biography . . . within the body in the muscles, organs even the bones and even in physiological rhythms."*
>
> **—Therese Schroeder-Sheker**

We "move in" to this building and expect it to serve us for a whole lifetime. We become so accustomed to the distortions and misalignments in our structure that our neurology actually realigns both cellularly and energetically with the new patterns. We are so malleable. We make it work. Until it doesn't. When the muscles are challenged this way and the bones are pulled out of alignment, we receive subtle warning signs that eventually speak louder and louder, almost to a scream. At that point we may be on the way to a hip replacement or knee surgery, or have disc issues, among other structural ailments. It is my intention to help you identify warning signs.

To see where this eventually leads, consider the number of older people who have migrated to the use of walkers. "How did I arrive here?" I often hear from my clients, "I never fell, I never broke a hip. I've just had years of enormous pain and I just could not stand on my legs over time." Their bodies have slowly become so twisted out of alignment that they can no longer carry themselves without support. You may not see yourself heading that way anytime soon, and I hope you are right, but unheeded aches and pains can escalate in ways you have not anticipated.

In my experience, for example, my sciatic pain was so intense and lasted so long I was terrified. Perhaps, in less obvious ways, your body too is distorted. Perhaps you have recurring pain or stiffness. Perhaps you can simply no longer do the things you once did with the same grace and ease. Perhaps your energy feels blocked or shut down. As we travel together through these pages, I invite you to become aware of the distortions in your own physical and energetic body, and then take a journey with me to unravel them, from their source.

Remember, we live in this body as a reflection of divine energy. I visualize divine energy as light. We are light in formation and we are informed by light. Energy is movement, cells vibrating with life force, excitement, and creativity. Looking into the eyes of a newborn we are reflected back with a knowing awareness that can only be divine essence. How does this "original" free untethered exquisite dancing movement become constricted, cloudy, and distorted—not only in our physical structure but in our emotional and mental belief systems? How do we get so very tangled up and so far away from this precious movement that is our life's juice?

Where did the distortion begin? As children many of us moved with abandon, testing the limits of our physicality, enjoying the freedom that only can be experienced in a body that is not tormented with limiting pain. Starting at a young age, we learn to ignore the little things—the twisted ankle, the falls, the twists and torques from sports injuries—because they just don't bother us too much. As we get older, there's the occasional knee pain, the back "going out," surgeries incurred over years, challenging pregnancies, accidents. All this and more lives in your body, and shapes your body, whether you can feel it or not. That does not include the emotional stress that your cells remember, and your cells remember everything, from your lifetime and those of your ancestors. Eckhart Tolle calls this "the pain body" and it houses much more than just the myriad of physical chapters we have journeyed through.

"The triangle is the world's preeminent symbol of divinity."
—**Michael Schneider**

The years go by, the drama in our lives seeps into the cellular story of our being, and we begin to get farther and farther away from the truth of who we are. We become fearful of embodying this truth with the richness and the juiciness of our birthright because we have shrouded ourselves in distorted perceptions that have insidiously become the fabric of our being.

In crises, both physical and emotional, not only does the outer structure of the body become twisted; the inner flow of divine energy is also challenged. When we live in our habitual patterns and distortions, we lose connection to our creative essence. When the energetic movement becomes blocked, we begin to feel imprisoned in this structure, suffocating as we attempt to take deep breaths. How can we *be* the truth of who we are when our physical home is so very challenged and the life energy is attempting to move through areas that are clouded, congested, or constricted? How must this block our creativity, our curiosity, our ability to fully live our purpose here on Earth and give our gifts exquisitely? Our physical forms are the embodiment of divine wisdom and as we free up the entanglements, the confusions in our musculature, to allow the light to penetrate and awaken us ever more to our divine path, we become whole. We become available to the light and we live in our essence. "We become essential," in the words of contemporary spiritual teacher Thomas Hübl. "When we are essential," he says, "we taste what being in the flow really is; a taste of the original movement where creativity is spontaneous and emergent."[1]

Coming home to truth, coming home to source, having the divine light of awareness and inspiration guide us is our birthright. Imagine that light, flowing from the divine source, along the sacred conduits of your physical design. Visualize those rivers of radiant intelligence informing your awareness. We are gifted the few precious moments of our short lifetimes to inhabit the body, and I believe it is our sacred duty to be respectful of and responsible for it.

RETURNING TO THE SOURCE: THE PERINEUM

So where do we begin in our journey to unravel the distortions that block our physical and spiritual energy? We must return to the source. Where did your journey of embodiment start? As divine energy, who you are has no beginning and no end, but as this physical form, you had a beginning. An embryologist once confirmed for me that when conception occurs and a new person is brought into this realm of physicality, the very first of the rapidly duplicating cells form a particular part of your anatomy: the perineal body. From there we emerge. The source of our embodiment in physical structure, when we emerge from the great sea of divine energy, is the site that becomes the perineum.

The perineum is a diamond-shaped structure located deep in the pelvic floor protected by the sacral bones, the pelvis.

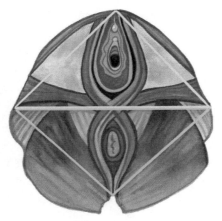

The Perineum

Functionally, the perineum contains structures that support the urinary, genital, and gastrointestinal viscera. These structures play a vital role in urination, defecation, sexual intercourse, and childbirth. The central point of the perineal area houses the perineal body, which is the place my teaching focuses on. Containing skeletal muscle, smooth muscle, and collagenous and elastic fibers, it is a point of attachment for muscle fibers from the pelvic floor and the perineum itself. In women, it is located between the vagina and the external anal sphincter, supporting the posterior part of the vaginal wall against prolapse. In men, it lies between the bulb of the penis and the anus.

"Expect anything worthwhile to take a long time."
—Debbie Millman

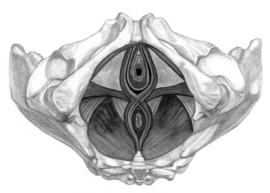

The Female Perineum

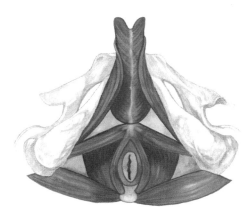

The Male Perineum

This particular domain of our anatomy—the pelvic floor—is still somewhat of a mystery to us. In Western industrialized societies we have shrouded this place in fear and judgment. It is also the focus of cultural taboos, sexual taboos in particular. While we have migrated through a myriad of shrouded secrets in these many years we have the cultural, historical information in our "warehouse" of cellular information.

Interestingly, other cultures have a different relationship to this area of the body. In yoga, the perineum is the site of the lotus flower, petals unfolding. In the Bhagavad Gita, a seven hundred–verse Hindu scripture (which is part of the Hindu epic the Mahabharata) Krishna is counseling Arjuna and engages him in a dialogue concerning the attainment of liberation. Arjuna has a very difficult decision to make and is deeply disturbed at what he is being asked to do to gain such enlightenment. To which Krishna at a place in the story, says that the seat of wisdom, knowledge, intelligence, is not in the mind; it is in the seat of the spine.

As a practicing yogi and teacher for many years I came to intimately understand what this means. The energy at the base of the spine, where all the nerves emanate from the spinal cord, to feed every organ in our body, must flow freely to allow us to be completely

"Our cells are formed in the intimate embrace of molecules receiving God the holy spark of life. They are sacred vessels for divine love . . . reflections of mystical teachings through the ages."

—Sondra Barrett, PhD,
Secrets of Your Cells

informed by the light. The cerebral spinal fluid flows through the central canal of the spinal cord and the four ventricles of the brain. A dear friend of mine, a cranial sacral practitioner, likened it to a garden hose. When that hose is twisted and torqued in a variety of places along the viaducts, the base is not fed; the journey in the river from the head to the base and back has many traffic jams and we become limited in the energetic flow to the organs.

Whether from our current lifetime's story or the inheritance of many lifetimes that came before, this place where the light of the divine lands within us has been compromised. Fear causes constriction, contraction, and a lifetime of behavioral patterns imprisoned in our cellular memory. Just as we literally "began" at the perineum, so does our physical distortion start at this same site: the perineal body, in the very center of the perineum triangle. The muscle fibers are stretched across, and spiraled around this space in so many convolutions, like a rubber-band ball. And, over time, these fibers pull, twist, and torque other fibers, ultimately distorting bigger areas that then pull on the attachment sites on the bones of the pelvis and the legs, twisting the bones out of alignment and contributing to urinary and prostate situations and more. This body is like an architectural structure and there is not one part of the structure that is not affected by the pulls and turns of another.

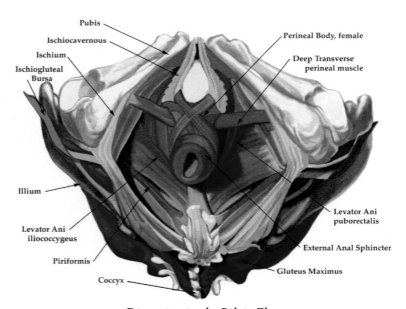

Distortion in the Pelvic Floor

As we begin our journey to unravel the distortions in our physical and energetic being, we begin again in the pelvic floor at the site of the perineum. To undo the contortionist patterns in this metaphorical rubber-band ball, we have to go into the original dysfunction at the "core" of the ball. Taking off one rubber band at a time from the outside in will not be enough. In the chapters that follow, I will be asking you to return, again and again, to this small but amazingly powerful physical location.

VISUALIZING THE PERINEUM

Let me introduce you to the basic anatomy of this area of your body. The pelvis is shaped like a bowl—the kind you might stir cake batter in. The two large pelvic (hip bones) and the sacral bones forming a protective home for the organs in the base.

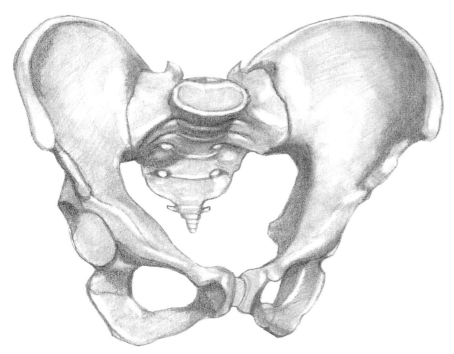

The Bones as a Container

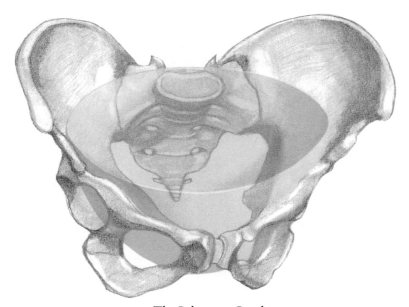

The Pelvis as a Bowl

The most helpful image I've come up with for the perineal body is a clock face. Imagine you are looking down from the crown of your head into your own body. Visualize the circular one-inch area between the anus and the genitals with a dot in the middle and numbers arranged around the perimeter. The point representing 12 o'clock sits at the front of the circle, behind the genitals, 6 o'clock is in front of the anus, 3 o'clock is on the right side of your body and 9 o'clock on the left.

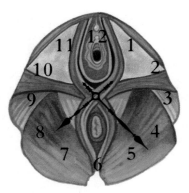

The Female Perineum Clockface

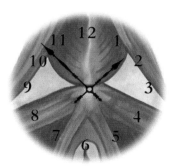

The Male Perineum Clockface

Now imagine energetic lines, like lasers of light, reaching from the center point out to every number around the circumference of the circle. Between these lines are numerous fibers, like the second hands of a clock, but multiplied countless times. There are a multitude of fibers between each and every number.

Perineal Body Enlightened

In a perfectly aligned body, the perineal clock lies flat, parallel to the ground, with all the numbers balanced at the same level and the fibers lying smoothly between them. Most of us, however, are not so lucky. Years of twisting and leaning to one side have distorted this area, twisting the fibers into misalignment.

Spend some time with this image and familiarize yourself with the idea that this little clock resides deep within you. You'll understand its purpose when we come back to the exercises in Part 2 of the book, and I will ask you to bring your attention to specific locations within the perineum by referencing the numbers on the clock.

BALANCE IN THE PERINEUM

Depending on how we have lived and played in this structure of ours, the alignment of the perineal area is not likely to fall dead center, with the perineal membrane lying across the center line between 3 o'clock and 9 o'clock, aligned perfectly. Here's another image I find helpful when thinking about this (as you're probably beginning to notice, I am a very visual thinker, and enjoy coming up with creative metaphors to help you "see" your own anatomy). Think of the perineal membrane as a seesaw board, like the ones you probably used as a child. Picture a tiny person sitting on each end of the seesaw, both of whom are the same size and weight. The board is therefore perfectly balanced, each of person's legs dangling evenly. Do you remember that feeling when you sat on a seesaw with a friend who was just about your same size, balancing in stillness?

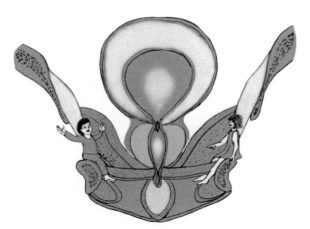

Perineal Membrane Balanced

As two-legged beings, the likelihood that the seesaw board across the perineum is perfectly balanced is small. When one side begins to have more power and the fibers are pulling across the perineum, the bones are going to be stretched more to that side and one of the little people's feet will be dangling closer to the earth, maybe even resting on the earth. Where does that put the person on the opposite side? And what do the fibers look like as they are being pulled, torqued, spiraled, and stretched across and downward? How do the bones respond? How do the organs respond?

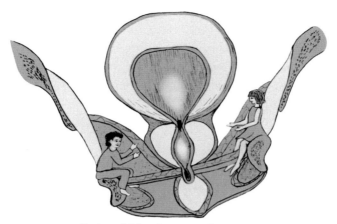

Perineal Membrane Unbalanced

I'll return to this seesaw image, as well as the clock, in the exercises in Part 2, where I will teach you how to bring balance and alignment to this part of your body.

JUDITH'S JOURNEY

Let's return to Judith, the artist whose creativity and energy was stifled by her pain-ridden body. In all the therapies that she had experienced over the years, no one had ever spoken with Judith about the perineal area. She had even gone to a pelvic floor physical therapist who, in her words, "performed" therapy on her but never ever said one word to her. Judith felt not only alienated from her own body but alienated from her therapists. Alone and bereft, she craved support and safety.

As Judith and I worked together for our first twelve sessions, we traced her struggle with balance, her several falls and mishaps, to her pelvic floor imbalance due to the misalignment of the musculature around her bones. Being pulled to one side, she was simply unable to use her leg bones as they had become imprisoned in the distorted musculature. Her leg bones could not reach out of the pelvis to support her back and like so many of us in this Western culture, she wound up with back stress.

Drooping into one side, her psoas muscle, which attaches to the inside of the upper thigh, was not able to elongate her legs. As this powerful muscle ultimately attaches to the lumbar spine she could not lift her upper body out of her pelvis. Like a long very thick rubber band, the psoas has such a magnificent job to perform for us. As it elongates the femur bone and stretches across the pubic bone, behind the pelvic bone, and emerges in the lumbar area, we are able to elegantly grow out of the pelvic floor in two directions.

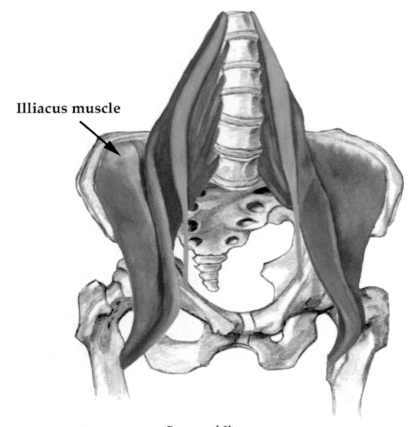

Psoas and Iliacus

For Judith, like most of us "two-leggeds," the muscles lying along the ver-tebrae, the erector spinae, did not have the support and space needed to elon-gate her entire spine. She kept collapsing more and more as the spaces became more and more constricted. With her energy unable to freely move, she began to collapse in ways that were not just physical.

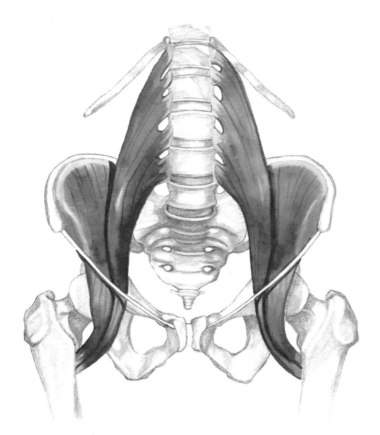

Attachment of the Psoas Muscle on the Vertebrae

As we began to journey through the distortions and ravelings of the muscle fibers in her legs and around her hips, Judith began to feel the deeper layers of constriction. Space began to expand deep in the pelvic floor and she could actually realize how out of alignment her pelvis was. At one point, she exclaimed, "That's why my knees are in such turmoil." Now she began to understand how she'd created her distortion, her unique map of entangled fibers. As she unraveled, she began to lift up out of her pelvis and extend her legs down into the earth. "I feel more elegant!" she said.

The shift Judith experienced was not just physical. She recognized how her pain had caused her to close in on herself, cutting her off from her creativity. As the muscle fibers released, so too did her passion for creating, and to her great joy, she began to paint again.

AN INVITATION TO EMBODY

The unraveling of the many stories of many lifetimes, of our "archeological" heritage and all of the journeys that have come before us is indeed an awe-inspiring task. Here we are in a body that has become challenged, tangled, raveled, and confused, and in pain and discomfort. As we unravel crystallized areas where there is reduced energy flow, we awaken to new ways of being that perhaps are now ready to inform us. Awakening is a profound path. When we are physically challenged, oftentimes we crawl off and allow the shadows of pain to inform us. It so much more of a challenge to choose to be informed by the light, to choose to flow in the divine river that connects us to source.

Be prepared, this journey will not be easy, especially for those of us who want to have the answers *now*. As the shadows emerge through the constricted areas, you may be asked to integrate that which perhaps you never even knew or did not want to know existed. But as you do so, you will also discover new potential, abundant possibility, new sources of light and energy. The fear that comes with prolonged pain, and the frustration that comes with not knowing how to deal with it, may be overshadowing deeper truths. Having tools to unravel the distortions may bring you into closer relationship with those parts of yourself that have been in a period of "rest" waiting for just the right moment to awaken out of a long sleep.

> *"We are architects of our experience."*
> **—Bruce Lipton**

I am humbled by what it means to "embody"—to live freely in the enlivened home we call our body and to make space for it to house the whole truth of who we really are. To embody, as I understand it, is to expand so dramatically that the energy coursing through our physicality, the light from our divine source, informs us as to who we really are. Do we have the courage to be truly embodied?

I love Andrew Harvey's concept of "radical embodiment."[2] Harvey, a scholar of religious and mystical traditions, beseeches us to awaken and embody our sacred nature so that we become true agents of change. Imagine what we could *be*, what we could *do, give, create*, if we were completely inhabiting this gift we have been given, if we were awake and aware of all that we are. We have been given amazing tools to complete the divine mission we are here for. For this we must have our physicality complete and whole.

I am in awe of the attention and focus it takes to undo a lifetime's distortion, in body and perception. Awakening is not often easy, perhaps never easy.

It is not comfortable. Yet living in a painful body, seeking remedies to put the Band-Aids on the pain, is not going to get us back to living freely.

This process is one that we must understand both in our mind intelligence and our cellular intelligence. We are familiar with the first, but in our culture, we have neglected the wisdom of the body and must relearn how to listen to what it is telling us. This journey—energetically, physically, emotionally, and mentally—is all about movement. It is all about stillness. It is about understanding our cultural lineage, our archaeological lineage, our familial lineage. It is about recognizing all we have unconsciously and consciously taken on from a myriad of sources. It is about honoring, acknowledging the path we are here to walk, the destiny that we are here to become.

As we embark on this journey, remember that it is not just a physical transformation. No longer can we look at this human form as muscles and bones, fascia, organs, and so on, without honoring and enlisting the energy body in our healing. How thrilling it is that we live in a time when we are awakening to the totality of our life form—all the way from the source of consciousness informing us and creating through this structure of our physical body. We are indeed a magical design. The intelligence of the divine energy will inform us at every step of the journey. Let us open the energetic pathways to move with freedom and joy. Let us explore the process of healing, come home to essentiality and original movement, and reclaim our birthright as energetic light-beings.

This journey we are on is far bigger than our physical pain, which of course becomes our main focus when we are in it, and the search to alleviate it. Resistance has become a learned pattern. We are here to *be* the light, informed by the light and live our destiny, our purpose here in this body. We have the ability to go back behind the distortions and expand into this never ending flow that we are a part of together. We are here to give and be generous. We are here to awaken and be responsible for the love we are.

Thomas Hübl likes to say that, "responsibility is the ability to respond."[3] In order to have that ability to respond to our sacred mission here in this world, we must have functioning bodies that can support us.

For further resources to support your inquiry, including videos, guided audio exercise, and more visit:

www.corebodywisdom.com

CHAPTER 2

READING YOUR BODY: WHY YOU'RE NOT STANDING ON TWO FEET

"I believe that the physical is the geography of being."
—Louise Nevelson

STANDING ON TWO feet: it is one of the defining features of our humanity. We are *hominids*—our upright stance distinguishing us from all but our closest cousins, the primates. And yet the truth is that most people are not really standing on two feet at all. My client Adeline knew this. Almost eighty, she was in a walker when I met her. "I feel like a one-legged person!" she declared.

Adeline did not understand why she could not rise from a chair or her bed without support. She never broke a hip, yet her physicians and physical therapists told her that she would ultimately have to get ready for a motorized chair. At that point, this very brilliant woman said, "No, I don't think so!"

She did not know how she was going to turn this around, at her stage of life, but she knew she would find out. That is when we met. Adeline heard that I work with people to regain the ability to stand in their leg bones, not just on their legs. That intrigued her and so we began.

As I watched Adeline leaning on her walker, demonstrating her challenges getting up from her dining room chair to retrieve something in the kitchen, two things struck me.

The first was her enormous zest for life. Here she was, encased in a physical story that did not make the slightest bit of sense for her. Her excitement for learning, teaching, and relating was so abundant, and the woman I could

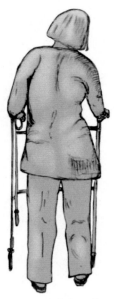

A Painful Walk

truly see within was not the woman struggling to rise from her chair. I could see her skipping down the hall, brilliantly moving towards her next amazing life episode. She confirmed my observation when she told me, "My body knows I'm eighty. I don't feel that way at all. It's like my inner four-year-old has come out to play and my body is confused!"

The second thing that struck me as I looked at Adeline was that her anatomy was not so different from that of most people, even those who are decades younger. Distortion, misalignment of muscle over bone, and imbalance prevents us all from standing on two legs!

You may not be aware of it, but in all likelihood, you stand more on one foot than the other. The distortions that are woven into the musculature of your body have left you out of balance, torqued, and unstable. We don't think we have much in common with someone like Adeline, whose legs cannot support her own body, but in fact the difference is one of degree, not of kind. Over my many years working with human bodies, I have developed the ability to see the imbalance, the distortion, the dysfunction in the structure. I'd like to teach you to do the same.

I'm sure you've had those moments when you're waiting to checkout at the supermarket or standing on a subway platform and you notice that you are resting on one leg, leaning to one side or the other. I was recently at the Department of Motor Vehicles getting a new license and the lines were very long. The array of postures I witnessed would have been funny had I not known that the discomfort these folks were experiencing was somewhat acute. Some luckily had a wall to lean onto. Finding balance— that central energetic line dispersing and distributing energy evenly so that we can just be present without rocking side to side—seems so challenging for most of us.

When we crawled on all fours as a baby, we used the limbs in a much more facile way and stretched the inner body differently. The baby's motion mirrors that of our ancestors. We walked on four limbs for a much longer time than we have walked on two. Our archeological history and lineage is embedded in our cellular, energetic memory banks.

Being on two legs is challenging. We have to rely on our lower limbs for much more, and gravity has us collapsing into the pelvis in a way that is not true for a four-legged creature. We have lost the sensory awareness of how to lift ourselves out of the pelvis and stretch the spinal muscles out of the pelvis. Anatomically, there is enormous stress put on the pelvis. We are constantly challenged to find balance, and the falls and mishaps that we have along the way continue to challenge this home of ours. Even our everyday activities present a challenge—standing, walking, cycling, running, carrying weight.

From the first steps we take as a child, we move into a most precarious position. The moment we stand upright, we favor one side over the other. As we grow, our bodies accommodate this imbalance, until it feels quite normal. Before we can begin the work of unraveling the distortion, it's important

"Nothing, of course, begins at the time you think it did."
—Lillian Hellman, Playwright

to be able to recognize the particular form it takes for you. Awareness comes before behavior change. We cannot move forward, free up the pelvic floor, and realign to create freedom until we know where we have been to create the distortion and confusion to become imprisoned in our structure. We must have enormous compassion for ourselves as we go through the unwinding journey home to original movement, a journey that will have you embarking far deeper than through distorted muscle fiber.

On this journey, there are many levels that you will learn to see, some of which are invisible to the eye. But the first level can be observed quite easily, standing fully clothed in front of a mirror. Let's take a look at your body and see if you can learn to recognize its particular patterns.

TAKE A LOOK IN THE MIRROR

There is a lot of important information you can glean about your own structure as you stand in front of a full-length mirror. You will be able to see the manifestation of years of wearing muscle over bone like you wear your clothing.

Looking at your body, let your eyes gaze over the hip area and upper thighs. Look at how the legs descend out of the pelvis on each side and how the upper torso "fits" on to the lower. You can do this exercise fully clothed. Your clothing hanging on your structure will mirror the musculature underneath. Most likely you will see that there is a noticeable difference from side to side. Your upper torso will drop onto the side that you are collapsing into. Your pelvis will not be aligned evenly and one side will be leaning over and into your leg. I call this "the droopy side"—not very scientific terminology, but quite an accurate description!

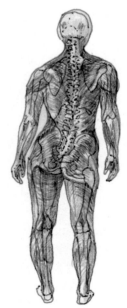

A Right "Droopy" Pelvis

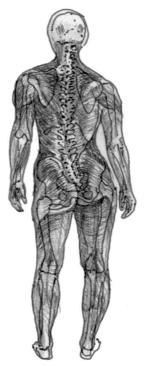

A Left "Droopy" Pelvis

Oftentimes, I have been told by clients that they have their clothing altered to accommodate their imbalances. "Oh yes, one shoulder is lower than the other and I have my suit jacket altered to handle that imbalance as the jacket hangs lower on one side," one gentleman told me, as if it was quite normal. That's one way of dealing with it, I suppose. Another informed me that "one leg is longer than the other and my seamstress alters the length to deal with that." I wondered if it were actually true. In a small percentage of the population, one leg is actually longer. For most of us, the upper torso is so dramatically collapsed onto the pelvic floor that the leg on that side *appears* to be shorter. In fact, it is jammed up into the pelvis due to the weight of the upper torso falling onto that hip and leg.

When you gaze at the very top of the thighs where they join with the bottom of the pelvis from one side of the groin to the other, can you see the fabric over your upper thigh wrinkling differently from side to side? Is the pubic bone lower on one side? Are you falling into one side of your body, drooping, collapsing on your leg? Do you have more weight through one leg more than the other? Which leg actually holds more of your weight?

Look to see how much space you have at the root of the thigh, which is the space between the femur bone (thigh bone) and the bottom of the pelvis. You should be able to palpate this space and feel depth, like a hollow, when the pelvis is in its correct anatomical position and you are not pushing the pelvis forward or tucking your "tail" under. If your pelvis is not aligned, however, you are most likely to feel tension, tightness, and lack of space. You'll be aware of the bulk of the quadriceps muscle lying on the femur bone and it will feel quite firm and hard under your fingers. This indicates that the femur bone is being pushed into the musculature.

Here's a funny image that I find helpful for understanding this anatomical distortion. Have you have ever squeezed yourself into very tight jeans and then spent an evening imbibing in food and drink? The stomach expands, and at the end of the night it isn't very easy to extract yourself out of the jeans in quite the same manner you poured yourself in! So you lie on the bed, unzip the jeans, and allow the belly to fall to the back side of the body, making room at the root of the thighs, where the femur and the pelvis meet. Then, with a little space you can inch the fabric of the pants down the leg and off. This is exactly how we must position the pelvis to have freedom at the top of the thigh.

Now, turn to the side and observe your posture. Is your sacrum—the lowest part of the vertebral column, where a long tail would attach if you had one—tucked under? A dog only has the tail tucked under when in a fearful stance. It is not that different for us. We do, in fact, have the remnants of a tail—the coccyx—and although considered a vestigial part of our development, I believe it is important to consider when feeling the pelvic anatomy. I find it helpful to imagine that historically, our "tail" was a long dinosaur tail trailing behind us. Imagine your own coccyx extending into a long tail.

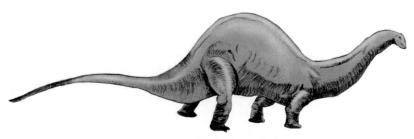

Dinosaur Tail Unraveled

Now, close your eyes and allow your internal gaze to travel deeply down into your pelvic floor. Feel the weight through your leg bones into your feet, into the earth. Now imagine you are resting in the bowl of the pelvis and looking up.

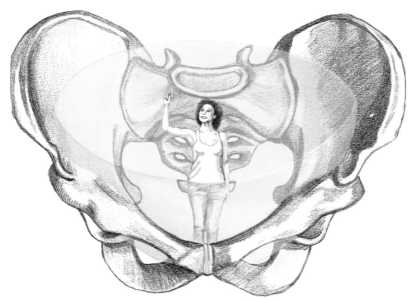

Living in the Bowl

When your eyes gaze up to your shoulders and the neck, what information are you getting? Are you evenly balanced across the upper torso, or is one shoulder lower than the other? Is one shoulder forward of the other? Are your neck and head leaning, turned, twisted to one side? Bring your attention back to the hips again, to your pelvic bones. Are you turning, twisting one hip around and forward to the other? Does that reflect into the upper body? Do the wrinkles in your clothing follow that movement?

Now look down at your feet. Are you collapsing one arch more than the other? Are your feet aligned so that the Achilles tendon is directly in line with the center back of the leg all the way up into the base of the buttocks? What can appear to be subtle differences—too difficult to see because we are so used to wearing our structure out of balance—produces dramatic results throughout the entire building.

THE NATURAL STANCE

Babies, when they begin to contemplate erecting, have a very cute stance, a natural posture. The diaper falls below the belly button, the nice round belly easily releases over the diaper and it seems as if the buttocks and the sacrum (the very base of the spine) are leaning back. When they decide that it is time to walk upright, they practice holding on to a table top or some stable structure, and then they wobble forward and back for a time to find that central line from which their center of gravity will inform them it's time to take off and walk.

It is not until we mimic the tall people in our lives that we become like those that came before us. I often look at a young child walking with a parent and both with the same droopy side and the same gait, the five-year-old mirroring his father's stance. I have often listened to clients report that they are starting to collapse into their "frame" and looking just like their parents—the rounded upper back with head falling forward, technically known as kyphosis, more often called the "dowager's hump."

You did not start out that way. Can you, right now, drop down into a full squat, landing on your heels, and feel complete freedom and comfort? No? You did it every day as a baby.

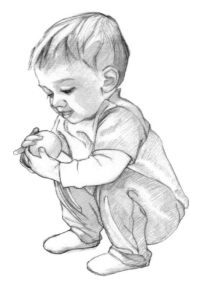

Our Squat Heritage

What happened? You changed the position of the pelvis in relation to the spine and the legs. Your center of gravity—your alignment through your base, up through the central channel of the spine, and up through the crown of the head—is completely off kilter. Hence, not only is it almost impossible to go all the way into a squat, but most likely your upper torso is falling forward over your knees and the weight cannot possibly drop down into your back body, through the heels.

Let's face it, as two-legged beings there are only so many ways that the spinal muscles can be challenged and become distorted. If we push the pelvis forward, which is the direction that we tend to do in Western society, then the bones have to respond in order to continue to support our structure. If something goes forward in the spine (the pelvis), then something else must go back. So we push the leg bones back, hyperextending the knees.

The thoracic spine (the upper-mid back in the area of the shoulder blades and below) rolls and collapses backward and the cervical spine (in the neck) rounds as well. What happens to the poor head, which weighs quite a bit (between eight and twelve pounds). It falls forward.

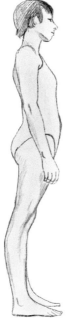

Hyperextended Knees

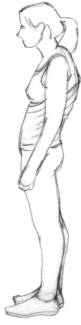

Distortion in the Spine

This puts tremendous strain on the poor cervical vertebrae at the base of the skull, those that protrude and sometimes ache when you are trying to hold your head up. Many clients have said, "How did I get this lump here?" I'm sure you have seen this posture on the street and in the marketplace again and again. You may look in the mirror and see this posture right now looking back at you. It might be subtler, but you can observe the signs even at a young age. I can feel the pain in very young children from having to carry that enormous backpack to school. And now we have a new term for a head falling forward due to constant cell phone use: text neck!

> *"Look well to the Spine for the source of disease."*
> —**Hippocrates**

Gravity has not been our greatest friend. We lose height as we sink into our pelvic bowl. If we push the pelvis forward and move the tail under too far, even a little bit so that the fibers are dragged from under the buttocks and upper thighs, coupled with the twists and turns, *we wind up* so dramatically distorted that over our lifetimes, we are no longer standing on two legs. In fact, we are barely standing on one. We are collapsed into the leg we favor and the upper torso is leaning down into it; there is no space at the top of the thigh between the femur bone and the pelvis.

This Western stance is also what leads our elders into walkers. People like Adeline find the walker a necessity because their legs are not properly aligned in relationship to the pelvis—not in the way necessary to carry this building for the number of years required to live healthfully in it. I find it striking that even those experts and practitioners who do pay attention to posture do not give enough attention to the position of the pelvis in relationship to the legs and the spine. The leg bones cannot release and extend out of a pelvic floor that is completely wound up. We need to release the bones, free them from the tight distorted musculature so that the legs can walk *through* the earth, not slide or shuffle on the earth. That is true weight bearing (something doctors tell us is essential for the prevention of arthritis)—creating space in the joints in order to have two legs to stand on.

We must stand *in* the earth, not on it. I tell this repeatedly to my students and the professionals I work with in a variety of body movement therapies. We are of the earth and the disconnect that we have experienced in relation to our presence on the earth mirrors the disconnect many of us feel with our own bodies. We have become separated from the energies that we are. We have looked outside of ourselves for the answers to our questions that are right here for us. We have been trained to not know.

In the story of the lack of freedom in the pelvic floor, structure and misalignment are rarely considered. When the pelvis is misaligned, all of the nerves that emanate from the spinal cord at the very base of the spine cannot possibly feed all the organ systems adequately. The effects of this are far reaching. In fact, in the book, *A Headache in the Pelvis*, Drs. David Wise and Rodney Anderson state, "It is our belief that most cases of chronic pain syndromes begin with a person's habit of focusing tension in the muscles of the pelvis. This tendency sets the stage for the disorder."[4] At one point in their book, which is a wonderful compilation of all the syndromes that arise in the pelvis, they note that destabilization of the pelvis is related to posture. "Typically, the pelvis has been tight for years, part of a default inner posture."[5] They add: "The tools of conventional medicine have failed to help muscle related pelvic pain in men and women … the muscles remain sore, contracted and painful in a self-feeding cycle of tension, anxiety, pain and protective guarding."[6]

My understanding, based on my own practice, is that this "default inner posture" is caused by a constriction that begins in the raveled muscle fibers at the site of the perineum. Years of contraction and distortion, moving all the way out to the outer layers. In this way, I make the connection between chronic symptoms in the pelvis and labeled "disorders," as well as spinal abnormalities that lead to bulging discs, need for hip and knee replacement and all other various and sundry structural problems that arise. In short, our pain is an *inside out* creation. How is it that most people in our Western cultures have scoliosis (curvature in the spine) in the sacrum?

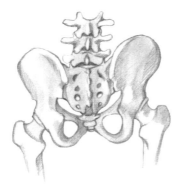

Scoliosis in the Sacrum

It makes sense when you consider that we are being pulled across the perineum from the very beginning of our movement journey as a child.

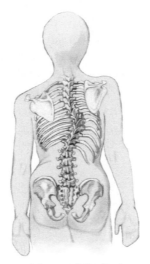

Advanced Scoliosis

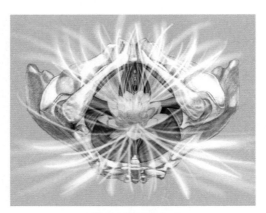

Light Unleashed

This may seem like an overwhelming predicament, a confusion that is impossible to undo. Surprisingly, though, awareness of anatomy is a wonder. When we take the pressure off the structure and make space, the *unwinding* begins and the rivers of energy begin to flow into the areas of congestion, awakening us to that original movement we once experienced, in our current life and in ancient memory. Like swimming in a river of light, the pelvic floor expands and the flow of energy, the intelligence held within the river, informs the spine and our entire being. We are awakening out of a deep sleep, one that we have imposed upon ourselves unknowingly.

OBSERVING INDIGENOUS PEOPLE

It is fascinating to me that people who grow up outside of Western culture, in indigenous tribes and societies that did not go through the industrial revolution, maintain a similar stance to our babies as they move into adulthood.

During my extensive travel over the years, I honed my sight and began to see the differences in posture amongst different cultures and more importantly across continents. When I was in Kenya and with the Masai and other tribes, I noticed immediately that the relationship of the pelvis to the legs and the relationship of the spine to the pelvis looked very different than they do here in America. How is it that huge jugs of water can be carried and balanced exquisitely on the head in some cultures? Right alignment is vital to this ability, since the smallest movement to one side or another has a dramatic impact.

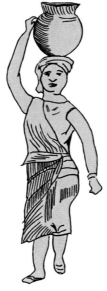

Balance and Beauty

The water jug on the head of the indigenous woman may look precarious, yet it is so balanced as to appear a part of the skeletal structure. If the jug were to weigh down heavily upon the skull, her entire spine would collapse. The sacrum would retreat forward, the tail sliding between the legs. The thoracic area of the spinal column would collapse backward, creating a huge convex curve and the legs would be imprisoned by the pelvis.

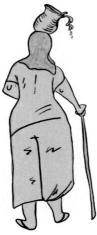

Carrying Weight Out of Alignment

Instead, she stands tall. She seems to be almost gliding along, and each step she takes is a movement created with the leg bones sliding freely out of an open pelvic floor deep into the earth. She is not walking on the earth, she is walking *in* the earth. She is not separate from it. An open pelvic floor allows her bones to reach deeply down and through, which allows her upper torso to reach that water jug out of her pelvis creating even more space. She is lifting that jug out of her pelvic floor as the entire spine extends up and out of the base. The muscles that extend the spine are free to do their magic. The power of the psoas muscle is unleashed.

The indigenous cultures carry themselves with an exquisite presence. The movement of these people's bodies clearly allowed me to see what "embodiment" is all about. They work very hard physically and their structure supports them with no effort so that as they run across the plains they are running with the support of the earth. They *are* the earth. They are not separated from the source of their sustenance.

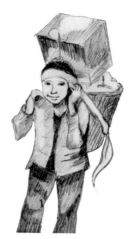

Lifting Up and Out of the Pelvis

The Sherpas in Nepal sometimes carry up to a hundred pounds in a basket on their backs, attached to the forehead with a leather band. They could not possibly carry that weight up the mountains with the pelvis pushed forward. It would slide directly down the back and onto the low back. However, as I watched them carrying their packs, I could see that the legs in relationship to the pelvis were slightly behind the pelvis. It was as if the legs reached out of open doors in the front of the pelvis to extend freely up the hills. The head climbing up and out of the torso was taking that heavy weight out of the pelvis as the head lifted up into the leather band, and it appeared to me that the sacrum was elongating down and out of the lumbar spine (the area directly above the sacrum, where those very thick vertebrae seem to create a whole lot of congestion and oftentimes bulging the discs in the L3 and L4 and L5 area).

Through my travels in Africa, India, and Peru, I saw people using their bodies very differently than we do in the West. They squat from the time they are babies, as we do, but they never stop!

Acupuncturist Esther Gokhale, aka the "posture guru," has been instrumental in helping thousands of people experience relief from back pain through learning from the "primal postures" of indigenous people. Her book *Eight Steps to a Pain Free Back* shows gorgeous pictures of indigenous people with their natural alignment. Her exercises recognize that posture is indeed a source of the misalignment and confusion that causes back pain.

In our quest to recover our natural posture, I think it is critical to begin in the deeper realms of the pelvic floor where the misalignment truly starts, at the site of the perineum. Outside-in fixes are not sufficient. Those of us who have visited chiropractors again and again in the hopes of becoming pain free realize that we want to take the pressure of the musculature off the bones. However, unless we delve into the source and unravel from the inside out, there is no amount of adjustments that will help to bring us back to original movement, to the original flow of our divine river, the tributaries feeding the organs and all of the vast network of our nervous system.

HOW HUMAN HISTORY SHAPED YOUR BODY

Our physical story, as I've explained, did not start with exercise that may have created an injury that spiraled into an avalanche of symptoms. Nor did it start with your immediate life story. We are each the updates of hundred of thousands of years of developmental and evolutionary history. Cultures for thousands of years have informed our ways of thinking, believing, and reacting. The culture, environment, and habits of previous generations have shaped our bodies, creating patterns with deep historical roots beyond our own lifetime.

For example, at the time of the Industrial Revolution in the West, human lives took an enormous turn. We began using our bodies in ways that did not serve our energy systems. Moving out of an agrarian world, we were now standing at machinery all day, which put enormous demands on our physicality. People now had jobs that demanded standing in postures for many hours that caused stress and tension on the structure. There was also more time to relax and enjoy the benefits of our hard work. That meant that we were sitting a lot more. Cars, couches, and chairs took us off the floor, the ground on which our ancestors sat and squatted, changing our alignment profoundly.

> *"The body is the crystallized past. It is the book we write from birth until death. All that we have ever done, felt, and thought is locked up in the body, the bones, the joints, the flesh. It is all there."*
> **—Dona Holleman, Yoga Practitioner**

I recall when I was instructing a teacher training program at my studios in New Haven, Connecticut, I invited an anatomy expert to speak to the class and she showed up with an actual bag of bones. That was a time when it was not easy to procure a human skeleton (but obviously still possible). She undid the heavily weighted muslin bag and ceremoniously laid the bones out on the studio floor with the care of a mother for a child. The assignment for our class would be to put these 206 adult bones back in their design and then analyze where this person had lived in the world, whether the person was male or female, how he or she used the body, what kind of work was engaged in, and what injuries redesigned the structure. In short, to read the life story of this human from the bones. This was, without question, the most fascinating time in my training course. I was an anatomy sleuth!

Years ago, when I began my study and research on alignment—or, rather, lack of alignment—in the human form, and how it wreaks havoc in the energetic system, I looked into anatomy books from the 1800s and compared the shape and form of the spine to the images in more recent books on the spine. I was fascinated to discover that the spines of years past did not have the dramatic curves that we now have in the thoracic and the lumbar. This confirmed, once again, that how we use our structure transforms the shape of that structure.

REINTEGRATING OUR HERITAGE

The osteopath, acupuncturist, and embryologist Philip Beach has made a connection between the natural postures of the world's indigenous peoples and the stages in the development of the human embryo. In his book *Muscles and Meridians: The Manipulation of Shape* Beach suggests there are what he has termed archetypal postures/movements that are inherently known in our cell structure. He states that, "Deep in our cellular memory we know these momentous processes, a massive momentum that binds us to the past." Our "modern lifestyles", he suggests, have "divorced us from a natural form of biomechanic self-correction with a resultant back pain that has become endemic in our societies."[7]

His understanding of spinal alignment is informed by his study of how the body developed in its embryonic form. He has peered into our embryonic morphogenesis—the biological process that causes an organism to develop its form and structure from the embryonic stage to the adult—and found it to be an encyclopedia of the processes we have all lived, experientially. "The genesis of one's basic shape is derived from these processes (cleaving, compacting, gastrulating, folding) that take place within the first six weeks post-conception, but shape continues to change during the course of a lifetime,"[8] he writes.

I met Beach several years ago, when we were both presenting at the 7th World Congress on Low Back and Pelvic Floor Pain. As we exchanged our professional wisdom, he provided the most wonderful validation of what I intuitively knew to be true: that the source of our spiritual embodiment in physical structure is the site that becomes the perineum. How the evolutionary spark embodies us and how we embody that spark to *become* who we are, embryologically, is completely fascinating to me. The two cells from the parents divide into eight. Embryologically, the perineum begins to develop after those first eight cells divide.

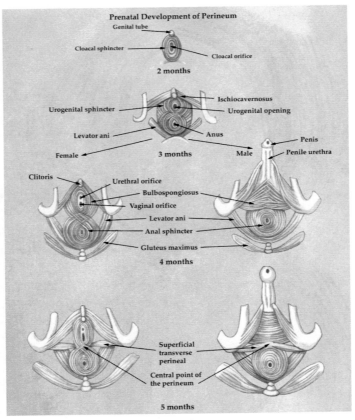

Our Perineum Beginnings

As the cells keep dividing, the embryo goes through what Beach calls "cellular choreography," a profound and lasting metamorphosis as the germ layers are formed. You might remember in your study of human biology the names of these layers: the endoderm (the deepest layer), the mesoderm (the middle layer), and the ectoderm (the outside layer). From this ectoderm layer, the skin, the nervous system and the eyes are derived; from the endoderm come the cells that line the gut from the mouth to the anus; the organs emerge from this layer. From the mesoderm, the perineum emerges, and from there, the vertebral column eventually develops, and the erector spinae muscles that support the spine; as well as muscle, bone, blood and the genito-urinary system. Beach likens this profound dividing and developing to a "physiological tsunami."[9] Our arrival into a structure is indeed a profound explosion in development. Just three weeks after conception all of this happens.

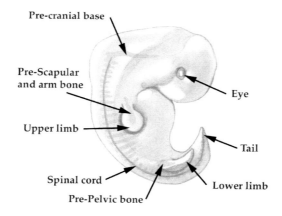

Pre-cranial base

Pre-Scapular
and arm bone

Eye

Upper limb

Tail

Spinal cord

Lower limb

Pre-Pelvic bone

Fetus at 5 weeks

The Fetus

On day twenty-eight, the limb buds emerge from the body-wall of the embryo as small buds that eventually and rapidly become large muscular structures. "Knowing how, when, and where they develop aids understanding and hence treatment of these complex structures,"[10] writes Beach. Back in 1759, a researcher, Casper Wolff, found a ring that is now called the Wolffian Ridge, which Beach describes as the ectodermal ring, that encircles the 4-5 week old embryo and "links the precursor tissues of the nose, eyes, and ears with the vagus nerve, the upper limbs, the nipples, the lower limbs and the genital tip into one cohesive interconnectedness at a critical stage in embryology."[11] All of the body parts touched by the Wolffian ridge "are of huge biological value and all come to be massively represented on the sensory cerebral cortex."[12] The fact that our sense organs are emergent from and connected to the pelvic floor is revealing. Our body is designed to be informed by our senses.

The early muscle cells that are pulled ventrally contribute to those that form around the pelvic orifices. This folding along the midline has the erector spinae muscles (those thick muscles that run along the vertebrae) twisting together to form the contractility that forms the muscular rings of the anal and urogenital cavities.

Beach was searching for a deeper understanding of human movement while working to help patients who came with low back, buttock pain, shoulder, neck, knee pain, and more. Informed by his research as an embryologist, he began to look deeper into our evolutionary heritage, studying the formation of the human structure through the evolutionary continuum of previous life forms to which we are related, such as the fish.

"Bones active, muscles passive; Bones leading, muscles following."
—Dona Holleman, Yoga Practitioner

Most interesting, he analyzed patterns of vertebrate movement and came up with what he calls the "contractile field" model. There are, he posits, "primal patterns that are embedded in our physiques. Each of these primary patterns of movement I call a contractile field . . . it is the interaction of the fields that creates coherent shape change."[13] These core mammalian movement patterns (flexing, extending, lateral flexing, twisting left and right, squeezing, pulsating, and peristaltic action) he believes, can be found in our evolutionary library. Amazingly, each contractile field embeds a primary sense organ.[14]

Beach is suggesting that in the study of movement we move our focus "away from groups of muscles based on body regions towards a whole organism perspective."[15] It is the relationship amongst the fields, he argues, that changes our shape.

For a more in-depth description of his field model of movement, you can dive into his book. Examples to reflect on include:

- Bending to the left and the right like a fish
- Bending forwards and backwards like a dolphin
- Twisting to walk and throw like a human
- Breathing like all mammals
- Limbs derived from a tetrapod (like a chimpanzee)
- A blood and food propulsion system like a vertebrate
- The fluid field, the common mediator to all movement. "In essence," Beach writes, "all animal movement is derived from the coherent manipulation of bodily fluids."[16]

He considers, for example, that the limb buds, emergent on day 28, are the originators of the developmental processes in the posture of the full-term baby that lead to sitting on the floor and then moving to a standing posture, then walking, and running.

The awareness of these contractile fields has supported my understanding of relationships such as that between the perineum and the jaw. Studying the embryological formation of the human, I now appreciate this connection in terms of misalignment and trauma. The upper palette in the mouth is very much the same dome shape as that of the dome shape of the perineum. When the pelvis is aligned, there is freedom in the jaw at the base of the ears. This has important repercussions for TMJ and other jaw-related problems

Beach proposes that it is our disconnection from these movement patterns, from our ancestral heritage over millions of years, that has us divorced from a wealth of information and an inability to self-correct. He connects this to the pervasive amount of back pain in our culture today. Based on this work, he has created an exercise protocol that he calls the "Erectorcizes," which guides people back into the postures that are associated with our ancestral heritage, reawakening cellular pathways that have become blocked.

The premise behind Beach's protocol is that our ancestors had the ability to "erect" rapidly in response to threats. The approach of predators was inevitable and demanded quick action. If you were an early human sitting around your campfire in a squat or cross-legged position, and a saber-toothed tiger was about to pounce from behind, you would quickly rise up onto the knees, and one foot then one leg would extend out ahead and you would run. Suddenly arising, standing down through the legs and rolling the spine up and out, came as second nature. That is what our structure is capable of doing, and still encoded in our DNA, although we may have lost touch with the ability.

I find it fascinating to turn the clock back in this way, to peer into our embryonic and evolutionary past. It is so informative to view our movement in the context of an enormous evolutionary palette we have inherited and continue to transform as we move. This is the reason for my continuing focus on unraveling the distortion beginning in the perineum. This is my motivation for helping you and others to create spaciousness in order to crawl out of the pelvis, and truly and honestly use your bones as they were meant to be used, in support of the muscles in divine movement.

THE FRONT BODY AND THE BACK BODY

There is one more important concept I'd like to introduce in our discussion of posture. We each have, in a sense, two bodies: a "front body" and a "back body." The space in between them is vast, although we mostly have no awareness of this. Because we are beings who wear our eyes in the front of the head, we focus forward and outward. We are always diving forward in our structure and negating the back of the body, the back of the heart. We generally do not take *all* of us with us in our awareness. We only partially embody our totality.

Picture yourself in a hammock, releasing into the fabric, being held so tenderly, trusting so much that you completely fall into the strongly woven mesh. There is no desire, no need to lift upward. You are completely supported. Your back body is sweetly letting go, and all the organs, all the internal parts of you, are falling back into the fabric of the back body, the hammock. That is where we are going on this journey. It is a journey into trust. If for years your body has been enslaved and imprisoned in the structure of distortion and pain, how can you trust that it will serve you and take you wherever you want to go and have been designed to go?

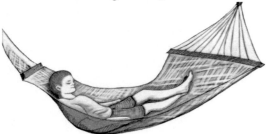

Surrendering into the Back Body

Our emotional pain, the shadows that we have kept tightly protected within the structure, within our cells, are keeping us from our true selves. Fear, shame, guilt, anger are all embedded in the tissues. Over time, as we unravel muscle off bone and free our inner being to be the divine expression of our truth, we can let go, we can fall back, we can trust. We can trust ourselves to fall into the divine being we truly are and create from a place of love.

This is a journey of the heart, and we must have compassion for the chapters that came before, that insisted we protect and distort. The history we now are becoming aware of is vast, connecting us to thousands and thousands of years of human unfolding. We are no longer willing to hide out and accept this pain. Here we are courageous heart warriors, coming home to that which is essential.

HOW DID YOU LEAVE YOUR BODY BEHIND?

Each one of us once had the body of the baby who could squat effortlessly to the floor. We were born with the cellular memory of our natural alignment. And yet, we find ourselves trapped in a distorted, challenged structure that can barely support us. Like my client Adeline, we may still feel like a little child inside, but our bodies will not allow us to move freely, joyfully, and with ease. How did we get here?

That was the question I asked Adeline. "How did you leave your body behind? When did the misalignment—physically, energetically, and spiritually—become so challenging that your body started to wear your story like clothing that no longer fits?"

"We are living our lives in only parts of our body. To really embody we need to make the journey inside whatever traumas, be they emotional or physical."
—Angela Farmer, Yogini

I wondered what life episodes from the very beginning of Adeline's embodiment had created the map for leaving herself behind. Accidents happen, traumas distort, beliefs attach like barnacles and create energetic logjams. Adeline's journey is not uncommon. The Qechua medicine people in Peru talk about "keeping secrets even from ourselves" and I now understand that we do so to protect ourselves from having feelings that were too painful. But these traumas, protected behind closed doors, deep in our cellular memories, create profound distortion in our psyche, our structure, and our spirit.

"When did I leave my body?" Adeline reflected on my question, and began to tell me her story. "I was always the scapegoat in my family. I remember being called names ever since I can remember. You're fat, you're fat." She scanned through the timeline of her life and focused in on a time fifteen years ago, when she was enduring ongoing traumas related to her son. She and his father divorced when her son was just five, and she pretty much raised him on her own. She admitted she was "very self-centered" and that she and her son were "way too close in those formative years."

> *"A person's ability to move is probably more important to his self-image than anything else."*
>
> **—Moshe Feldenkrais**

"He was all I had," she went on. "I was afraid of growing up, very withdrawn. I couldn't relate to people until I went to OA (Overeaters Anonymous). I didn't really know how tightly wound I was, inside and out. Around fifteen years ago, a therapist of my son's told me I was too involved in his life." Adeline recognized that her focus on her son provided the perfect "out" for her not to be fully in her own life. "I hid behind his overalls," she says.

I could hear and feel the sadness in Adeline's structure, as in her heart, as she continued her story. "My mother died in the early nineties. I was sixty-five and the loss and the grief was staggering." She paused, and then, as if an afterthought, after a long silence, a remembrance emerged out of the shadows, "Oh, and I had breast cancer after she died. I was glad she wasn't there to see me go through that."

Around this time, Adeline remembers beginning physical therapy. She couldn't remember exactly why she went—perhaps her legs were weak, or maybe her whole body—but it only made her physical issues worse. "When I first started it was because of IT-band weakness on my right side. Apparently I was wobbling and limping for quite some time without realizing it. I had what was called a Trendelenburg gait." (A Trendelenburg gait is a condition in which, due to the weakness of the hip adductors, mostly the gluteal muscles on one side, the body is unable to stand evenly on both legs and one side of the pelvis drops. The upper torso collapses onto the dropped side. This can also be caused by hip disease.)

After her knee replacement, Adeline was told she had a spinal stenosis. "Now I had learned it was something serious!" she says. "My previous doctor said it was only arthritis." She had a knee replacement, but woke up from knee surgery feeling the same pain in the same place as before. "The problem," she explains, "was the bursa (the small fluid-filled sac that cushions the knee joint) in my left knee responding to excess pressure because of the IT-band problems on my right side." She listed many different protocols she had tried, with little effect.

As Adeline relayed the chapters of her ongoing distortion, there was clearly a new self-awareness emerging from her storytelling. She had connected more of the dots in her lineage and in her history. But it was hard for her. "I can't bear thinking of all the misery I endured," she told me.

When Adeline talked about her breast cancer, it was clear it was a formative time in her life. "I did have amazing supportive friends ferry me across that milestone. My spiritual community really turned out for me when I had my breast surgery. I asked! They were so kind and giving. I needed a ceremony for healing and I was gifted one. Before I went into surgery my friends and the surgeon gathered in ceremony. Ten days after surgery I was in my tai chi class."

I could "see" and feel the layers of her story emerge. Adeline carries the years of distortions, in body, mind, and spirit. Awakening is tender and we are so vulnerable as the caretakers of this being we have been gifted.

Gradually, she said, "I became more of me, instead of the shy more depressed me. I had grown enough to know what I needed and how to provide it and ask for the support of others." I could feel her gratitude and growth from the child who had retreated to the woman I know now. The tenderness in her voice and the release in her body were sweetly and softly emerging.

"All those years where I had to forget who I am to protect myself, hide out with overeating, live in fantasy and illusion, are behind me now, yet they have informed me." She reflected: "I have been so unconnected to my body but over the years have become more connected. Now, I see myself like a seedling that carries all the possibilities for life. Yes, my four-year-old has indeed come out to play!"

Adeline could only look deeper into the origins of her pain when she felt safe enough to feel the truth of the mechanisms she used to hide from it—her overeating, her dependence on her young son, her development of behaviors

> *"Health is not something you pursue and get . . . it's something that you already have until you disturb it."*
> —**Dean Ornish, M.D.**

that would allow her to survive as a young single mother. Terrified of feeling her fear, she put those feelings in places that could only fester and come out in other ways eventually. She could not have received her own painful story and allowed the terror to be felt. The stakes of survival were too high. She was not ready. The pain in her body was sequestered deep in the tissues of her every cell, defining and redefining her structure. Only when she was told she would be ready for that motorized chair and had garnered years and years of support could she say, "No." Her own small voice, protected deeply inside as a child, clearly called out. When we can say *no* to other voices that want to control us and *yes* to ourselves from that place of deep safety and belonging, we are ready to become more of our innate divine truth. Adeline was made ready!

Adeline's situation is not unlike so many others. People are seeking to find the source of their discomfort many "conditions" later. I have enormous compassion and empathy for this vulnerable condition we find ourselves in where we are continuously seeking the answers and we just do not have enough information to be informed participants in our own care. Let's continue on our journey and learn more about our own anatomy, so that we can become our own healers and release our true essence into the world.

For further resources to support your inquiry, including videos, guided audio exercise, and more visit:

www.corebodywisdom.com

CHAPTER 3

THE ANATOMY OF DISTORTION

"Movement never lies."
—Martha Graham

IN THIS CHAPTER I want to focus on the "meat of the story"—muscles and bones. If you observed yourself in the mirror, as I suggested in the previous chapter, you will have begun to see your own imbalances reflected on the surface of your body—your posture and even the wrinkles in your clothing. Now, let's go a step deeper, looking below the surface of your skin at the musculature and the bone structure beneath. We'll focus on the hows and whys of your own anatomical design, to educate you as to how this distortion evolved, a distortion that ultimately created enormous confusion in the physical and energetic fields.

How we create the pain cycle, physically and emotionally, is vital information in our healing. For this chapter let us delve into the physical dimension: your anatomy. While I want to provide you with as much information as I can to help you be an informed participant in your own healing process, I will attempt to be as "gentle" in my descriptions as I can. This is not meant to be a crash course in human anatomy, but rather, a window into your physical structure that supports your ever-awakening consciousness about how your personal distortion evolved.

As you begin to unravel and awaken to the source of your dysfunction, you will become more informed and can begin to create a deeper relationship and understanding with your own body. My intention is for you to take ultimate responsibility for your own healing. To do that, you must have the knowledge of how you arrived here.

What I have learned, from working closely with hundreds and hundreds of bodies and witnessing many more in large workshops, is that this design is indeed individual to each one of us. The way we have inhabited our bodies, worn the muscles over our bones and created this saga of distortion is indeed of our own design. Not one of us has lived in our body in exactly the same way. The exercises we do, the way we stand, walk, sit, lie down, are all causing muscle to stretch and ravel over and around our bones in a particular way.

HOW EXERCISE DISTORTS THE BODY

We are a culture that values exercise, and we love our sports in all their wonderful variety. We are also a culture that desires results very quickly. We focus on where we are going and most often negate and prefer not to know where we have been as the residue is often disturbing. We push on. We push through. We demand that this body perform for us.

There is no doubt that my generation, the boomers, were not going to give in to aging without a fight. In fact, we are the generation that was determined never to age in a debilitating way. Our kids would not put *us* in some nursing home! We attacked exercise, but, in our ignorance, we often did so with a misaligned structure. We took up running, tennis, biking, the hiking, yoga, dance, golf, climbing, and more—all such wonderful physical disciplines but difficult for a distorted body to handle. We propelled ourselves into the fitness world like we did the rest of life, with a passion to consume everything possible and become everything possible. Balance was not exactly our forte. The fitness revolution became a program that we fought to conquer, overriding the history that we carry in our cell structure, in our musculature. This "outside-in" approach, trying to impose fitness upon the body rather than unravel from within, became habitual.

Over the years, our forms of exercise have exacerbated the distortions already designed within our musculature. As we forced ourselves to push through, we created further imprisonment in our own design. We ended up locked in distorted structure, physically, emotionally, mentally, and spiritually.

Let's take a closer look at some popular forms of exercise and their effects on the body. I myself started out as a yoga practitioner, so this is one field with which I'm particularly familiar. According to Yoga Alliance, in 2016 36.7 million Americans (or 15% of the adult population) practiced yoga.

There were 52,746 yoga teachers registered with them, and undoubtedly tens of thousands more.[17]

Yoga has deep roots in Indian culture, where it was as much a spiritual practice as a physical discipline. The practice of yoga, the practice and refinement of the asanas (poses), is intended to cleanse and prepare the body for higher states of consciousness. However, in the United States we tend to approach yoga as a sport and, like in other sports, we attack to win. I have witnessed students pushing through pain, again and again, with no awareness of the necessity to go deep within first, to slow down and deepen their attention. You might think that yoga would help with our misalignment, but if the distortions are not addressed first, the poses can simply create intense anomalies. Yoga creates havoc for those who practice without awareness. When the pelvis is out of alignment, yoga does not have a foundation. Once we align the pelvis and begin to create yoga's ancient beautiful postural designs from an inner open pelvic floor, the practice becomes truly majestic.

Dr. Raza Awan, a sports injury specialist who uses yoga for rehabilitation, noticed that there was not much information available about yoga injuries, so he started tracking the data. "If someone is too flexible and gets into the end range of a pose without good support and muscle stability, it can cause wear and tear on joints," he observes.[18]

William Broad, science reporter for the *New York Times* and author of the controversial book *The Science of Yoga: The Risks and the Rewards*, in his research on hip pain and yoga, interviewed Drs. Jon Hyman, an orthopedic surgeon in Atlanta, and Brian T. Kelly, an orthopedic surgeon at the Hospital for Special Surgery in Manhattan. Dr. Hyman stated that he sees a relatively high incidence of injury as a result of participating in a yoga practice and that he does not see this in other modalities. Dr. Kelly voiced similar concerns. Yoga postures, he said, tend to throw hips into extremes.[19]

Let's take a few other examples. Golfers who twist repeatedly, unaware of the design of their muscle fibers, are creating more and more distortion with every stroke while bypassing areas of stress and tension. And as the golfers focus on the ball with each stroke, their head swings out of a misaligned pelvis, leading to herniated cervical discs. Hip and knee replacements, lumbar disc challenges, and rotator cuff problems are all associated with repetitive movements. Unaware of his or her internal design and the way it is inducing stress, the golfer pushes on to win the next game, to challenge his previous score.

The same is true of other athletes and performers. Runners, with a pelvis out of anatomical alignment, load more stress on a quickly moving body. Training for the next marathon, they pound the pavement with their zeal to reach the finish line. There are so few runners who allow the body to run them! Few have learned how to free the legs and torso from the pelvis to fly in freedom as they run.

Dancers tend to dance through their pain, whether the pain comes from dropped arches, spinal twists, or other common ailments. Basketball players perfect that beautiful jump shot, and football players make yet another astounding run to the goal, overriding the blows the body takes. Look at our sports heroes as they have aged and the results on their bodies.

While they are by no means all exercise-related, the numbers of people having hip and knee replacements in the last years are staggering. At the 2014 Annual Meeting of the American Academy of Orthopaedic Surgeons, it was reported that total knee replacements increased by 120 percent in the period from 2000-2009. When those numbers were further broken down by age, they showed an increase of 188% in the age range 45-64, and 89% in the age range 65-84. For total hip replacements the increase was 73% over the same period (123% in the 45-64 age group and 54% in the 65-84 age group.) These figures translate to 2.5 million Americans living with an artificial hip and 4.7 million with an artificial knee.[20]

As osteoarthritis is on the rise dramatically as well, it is believed that degenerative arthritis has a major role to play in these numbers of surgeries. The numbers of more physically active people are growing exponentially and the wear and tear on the musculature is the cause of this arthritis. According to Dr. Mark Pagnano, head of the Orthopedic Department at the Mayo Clinic, "the number of patients who are candidates for hip replacements at a younger age are growing."[21]

Thirty years ago it was common to have joint replacement occur in seventy-year-olds. Now there is a field of practice where orthopedic surgeons are specializing in arthritis in the young adult, and hip and joint replacement is performed on those as young as 25. According to the national Joint Registry 2012 Annual Report, knee replacements grew to 676,000 in 2009. If these trends continue, an estimated 600,000 hip replacements and 1.4 million knee replacements will be carried out in 2015. It is estimated that by 2030, the number of knee replacements will rise to more than 3.4 million. At Washington University and Barnes-Jewish Hospital a Young Adult Hip

Preservation Program has been established as there are so many young athletes developing arthritis and on the way to hip replacements.[22] Hip structural abnormalities are not considered when a young person takes on sports, though more have developed arthritis and are on their way to replacement surgeries so the issue is impossible to ignore.

Dr. Jeffrey N. Katz, professor of epidemiology and environmental health at Harvard School of Public Health and director of the Orthopedic and Arthritis Center for Outcomes Research at Brigham and Women's Hospital, has this perspective as a surgeon: "Young active people who are being slowed down in their lives are increasingly open to having these procedures." However, he does not see this so much as a "throwaway mentality." Rather, he says, they "have things they want to accomplish and they don't want their knees to get in the way."[23] This way of looking at the body as a tool to "get things done" separates us from the deeper truths of what we are here for.

So is exercise "bad" for us? Not at all. We are made to move, and athletes, at their best, are incredible specimens of how we can design a body to perform to perfection. I witnessed this as I watched the Masai warriors run across the plains in Kenya. They were a vision of beauty—the long spear held in exquisite alignment along the length of the spine as the legs seem to run backwards out of the pelvis and the upper torso run forward.

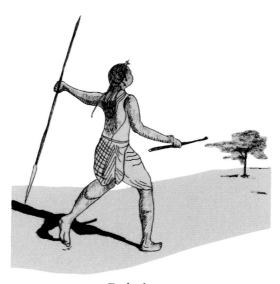

Embodiment

The key is to understand that exercise rests on the foundation of alignment, and if we do not take care to align the body first, the exercise will inevitably increase distortions. (In chapter 12, I will return to the topic of exercise and offer guidance on how to safely engage in the physical activities you love.)

ALIGNMENT, ALIGNMENT

A cookie cutter approach to your physical structure will not be enough to undo the distortion and bring you back to original movement. You need to understand how the activities you have engaged in have shaped and distorted your body. You may not immediately be aware of them, because the body is wonderfully adaptive. It does the best it can to work around the challenges we place on it.

Years ago, when I was taking a course at Stanford that incorporated dissection, I noticed something in the femur bones that startled me and had me in a quandary. There were small cuplike grooves along the length of the femur bones. I queried my professor as to what they were and why they were aligned so differently on each thigh bone. His answer was not satisfactory and left me confused for many years. What I discovered, years later through my own unraveling process and after witnessing the misalignment of the pelvis in relationship to the leg bones in most of my clients, was that these grooves are a result of the femur bones being thrust forward into the quadriceps muscles. The muscle fibers, which are having to hold on to a structure that is quickly moving out of alignment, must adhere to the bones in any way they can. They have to be creative, that's for sure.

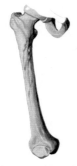

The Effects of Misalignment

Ah, alignment, alignment. The relationship between the pelvis, the legs, and the spine is so critical. The muscle fibers, which I liken to tentacles, attach deeply into the bone to attempt to hold the body up in some form of integrity as we twist, torque, thrust the pelvis forward, and wind fibers ever more firmly to the bones. This body, you can begin to see, is constantly doing the best it can to be upright. I marvel at how well the structure actually does over eighty, ninety years, and more. However, as we have all seen, there are a variety of postural challenges that we witness in others and experience in ourselves.

The journey back to freedom, to original movement, to experiencing the natural flow of energy can be a most challenging one, especially for those of us who tend to want answers and fixes *now*. Clients come to me who have been through the medical system, and oftentimes had surgery, but still need to unravel the distortion from the source of the injury, the congestion. I see light bulbs flash in their awareness when they realize that the twists and torques that preceded the dysfunction were all there as a precursor to the accident's results. Rolling the clock back and beginning to feel old patterns that settled in, early on, begins to inform us in the present time. Shadows emerge out of the space and time continuum and we become freer and more whole.

LEARNING YOUR PELVIC ANATOMY

I want to start by introducing you more intimately to your pelvic girdle and your pelvic floor anatomy. Remember, in chapter 1, I described the pelvis as best visualized like a bowl that you would stir cake batter in.

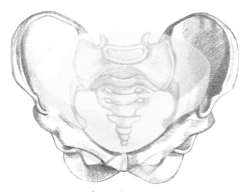

The Pelvic Bowl

It consists of the bones of the pelvis, which are the two hip bones (innominates), the sacrum and the one or two bones that form the coccyx (tailbone), and the two sacroiliac joints, the sacrococcygeal and the pubic symphysis. The sacrum comes from the Latin word, *sacer,* and by the Romans *os sacrum.* In many indigenous and ancient cultures, this bone has been known as the "sacred bone" as it supports the source of creativity.

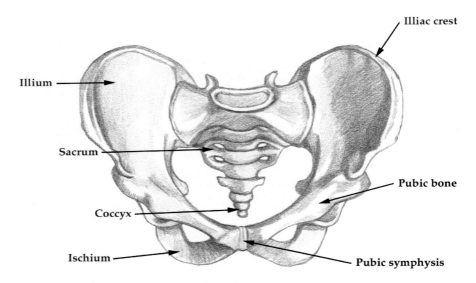

The Pelvic Bones

Harrison Fryette, a doctor of osteopathy writing in the 1950s, credits the "ancient Phallic Worshippers" for naming the base of the spine the "sacred bone." It's little wonder they did so, he writes, for "it is the seat of the transverse center of gravity, the keystone of the pelvis, the foundation of the spine. It is closely related with our abilities and our disabilities, with our greatest romances and tragedies, our greatest pleasure and pain."[24]

The pelvic cavity is surrounded by this bony structure and houses the reproductive organs and the rectum and supports the abdomen and these organs in the lower pelvis. It also provides the connection between the thorax, the lumbar spine, and the lower limbs. The pelvic floor is below this pelvic cavity.

For our study here, I want to focus on the perineum and the base from which we began our development. It is here, I believe, that the source of a lot of the distortion emanates from and you must be aware of the enormous complexity that is housed in this area. Once again, the perineal body in the center of the perineum, that approximately one-inch area located between the anus and the genitals, is the core foundation for understanding our imbalance. This is the spot where I draw the image of the clock face.

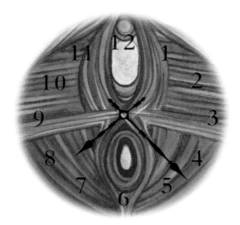

Female Clockface

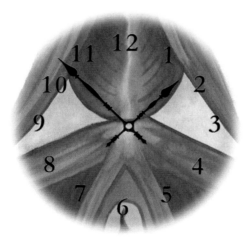

Male Clockface

It is helpful to refer again to the image of this pyramid-shaped area with the perineal body in the very center.

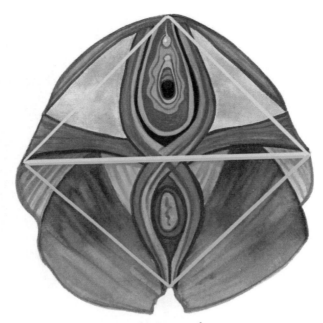

The Pryamids

This area that I want you to be aware of and focus on is the central part that is literally the source of our beginning in our human embodiment.

It may be difficult to conceive that this small one-inch area in the center of the perineum—the perineal body—is where we emerged from and the area from which our deepest distortion evolves. Deep in the pelvic floor resides the source of not only physical but of emotional pain. This place of our beginnings, of our light "landing" in this embodied form, is the deepest place of shadow, constrictions, and contractions.

Your assignment, so to speak, is to create a visual connection with this area. The places where we feel physical pain may be the result of deep emotional tensions that cause us to contract and distort muscle over and around bone. What does the earliest experience of fear, of not belonging, of lack of freedom, of not feeling safe, even in the slightest amount, create in the musculature? What effect do these contractions have in preventing us from fulfilling our sacred destiny here in this divine body? How is it that we are pulled and torqued and misaligned by these muscles? It starts from the first steps we take as a child and the pattern continues to evolve over all the years we use and misuse the body.

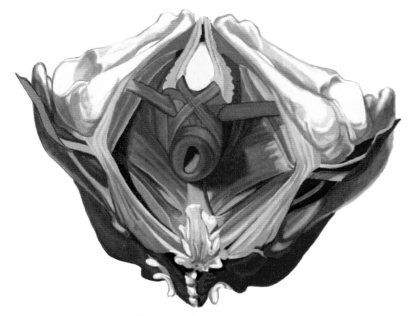

Distortion in the Musculature

Looking at the image of the perineum and all the muscle fibers that are stretched and skewed across this one-inch-plus area and connected throughout the entire perineal body, you can begin to get a visual picture of the confusion within this most sacred space. These fibers are connected across the perineal area and throughout the entire pelvis, behind the pubic bone and the sacrum and attached further out to the bony structure of the pelvic bones and out to the legs. We are being pulled and distorted with every step we take due to this original imbalance. Then we put another enormous stress on the structure with intense sports and perhaps even more when we lift something or just bend down to pick something up off of the floor. Because of the internal twisting of the muscle fibers pulling us further out of anatomically correct posture, a disc becomes challenged, or a whole host of other stories manifest.

THE MANY RAMIFICATIONS OF PELVIC PAIN

Chronic tension, holdings, contractions, and fear in the pelvic floor contribute to a host of painful symptoms that affect a growing population. According to a Yale University School of Medicine publication, twenty million people are suffering with bladder control problems, urinary incontinence, and chronic pelvic inflammatory disease (PID).[25] Chronic pelvic pain syndromes are estimated to be responsible for a direct health care cost estimated at $880 million per year. The list of symptoms associated with chronic pelvic pain syndrome (CPPS) is extensive and includes pelvic floor dysfunction, prostatitis (bacterial and nonbacterial), levator ani syndrome, vulvodynia (vulvar vestibulitis), urethral syndrome, pelvic floor myalgia, pudental nerve entrapment, and interstitial cystitis (IC). Along with these symptoms and syndromes, incontinence and bowel and sexual dysfunction oftentimes play a major role. To say that people caught in this cycle are debilitated is an understatement.

Drs. David Wise, PhD, and Rodney Anderson, MD, in the Department of Urology at Stanford University, creators of the well-known and well-researched protocol on CPPS—formerly known as the Stanford Protocol, now called the Wise-Anderson Protocol—claim that the old forms of treatment, drugs, and surgeries, were not addressing the complexity of this syndrome. They consider that "muscle-based pelvic pain is a condition in which mind and body meet in the pelvic floor,"[26] and focus on rehabilitating a chronically tight pelvic floor, "...and at the same time stopping the nervous system arousal that feeds pelvic floor tension."[27]

One of my clients, Ajay Narayan Patel, was like a walking catalogue of these pelvic syndromes. When I first met him, by chance in a cafe in Berkeley, California, he had placed a special cushion on his chair (a cushion that I later learned he carries with him by bicycle everywhere he goes) and I could see that he clearly was in pain in his pelvic floor, back, and more.

I wanted to know how he handled his pain. It turned out that Ajay, a professor who was forty-two years old at the time of our meeting, was a patient of Drs. Wise and Anderson at Stanford. He was not shy about letting me know about the severe pain, the incontinence, and the bowel and sexual dysfunction that he had been suffering with for years. At his young age, he was already crippled by back and pelvic pain, and oftentimes had to be carried up stairs when he taught. He could not travel by plane or car, stand in front of a class, or engage in sexual relationships.

Ajay's story goes much further back—a veritable A to Z of syndromes and symptoms, spiraling one into the other. On top of all that, at forty years old when picking up a podium his back "went out." He described the pain as "electrical waves like a tsunami that surged throughout my back." A few years later, attempting to pick up a bookcase, the same pain radiated throughout his pelvis, the sacrum, the lumbar, and his pelvic bones. And six years after that, diabetes and high cholesterol were added to his list of woes. His immune system was taking him on a downward spiral, and his physical, emotional, and spiritual being were barely hanging on.

Ajay is one of the most extreme cases I've ever encountered, but he is also deeply committed to living the fullness of life as an active participant in his profession. Despite his list of medical "syndromes" he has the ability to draw on his abundant zeal for life to get him through. He is an ardent student and researcher, dedicated to being the best client/patient to learn and practice what will inform his being and allow him to heal and live more passionately. As an avid cyclist, he can always be seen riding through the streets of Berkeley, sitting in an anatomically correct posture that gives him some relief. He swims almost every day, has completely transformed his eating plan, lost many pounds, and is truly invested in seeing this world we live in be "better."

"If weight is habitually never transferred through the center of a joint, some of the muscles that cross the joint are constantly being stretched while others are more contracted and unable to stretch as much."

—Irene Dowd

On Ajay's journey through pelvic floor research, he has discovered he is experiencing pudental nerve entrapment, which is the compression of the pudental nerve. It has not been easy to ascertain that this is the mystery behind all of his pain. The enormity of muscle fiber in the floor of the pelvis with various injuries to the low spine and other challenges his body experienced caused the distortion of muscles, tendons, and tissues.

I am deeply humbled and honored to coach Ajay on his healing journey, knowing that he is coaching me too, as we travel through the distorted layers, both physically and energetically.

After just two sessions, Ajay began to experience some relief and after eight, began to incorporate his new awareness into his daily regime of exercises. At one point, with such vulnerability, he looked up at me and said, "Ginny, I just may fall in love again." As I write these words Ajay has taken a semester off from teaching, dedicated to transformation with more hope than he ever thought possible.

It is my understanding from all my years of working with clients that our structure has everything to do with the stories that evolve. We are in a constant fight-or-flight mode, sucking up, sucking in, winding, raveling, and distorting. We are unaware of the dark shadows that have contributed to our way of living and push us forward into the next imbalanced version of ourselves, all the while unaware that we are leaving our real selves behind. As we take the pressure and tension off the musculature, places of constriction unwind creating space. Energy moves and hidden feelings emerge out of old rooms, rooms we have previously closed in order to protect ourselves from feeling the source of an original hurt. Our journey to wholeness, to becoming free in body, is more than a physical one.

The muscles of the pelvic floor are quite complicated and an amazing design, such that if we are out of anatomical alignment these muscles are all called into action in a negative way. "Arranged on top of each other like roofing tiles that form a funnel"[28] writes Eric Franklin, in his informative book *Pelvic Power*— an excellent reference for understanding the pelvic floor and diaphragm.

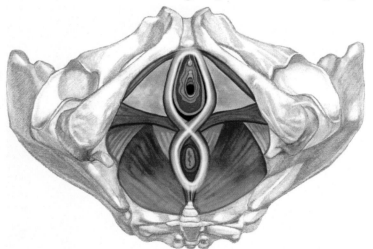

The Figure 8

The perineal triangle has three muscles on it that form the outer layer of the pelvic floor and there are two more triangles lying on the bigger triangle. There are layers upon layers, and the distortions, the torqueing, and the pulling associated out to the bony structure are intense. Also, it's important to realize that the muscles are all associated around the vagina, attaching to the clitoris, and the penis, and into the anal sphincter, creating a "figure eight" of muscle fibers. At the center where the lines of the figure eight cross is the small one-inch-plus area that is the source of our beginning.

Extending to either side, out to the bony structure of the pelvic bones, is the larger perineal membrane, which ultimately pulls on the bony structure and distorts the bones.

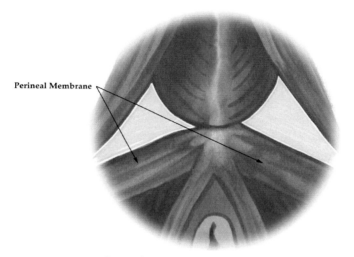

The Male Perineal Membrane

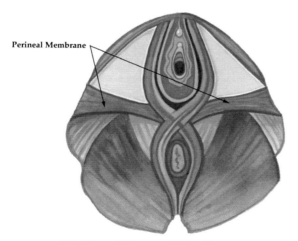

The Female Perineal Membrane

Collapsing into one side of our body, dropping into one leg so that the flow of energy is reduced, we are barely able to extend either leg out and into the earth, setting the stage for pain and dysfunction. Achieving freedom in the perineal center and entire perineum area allows the rivers of energy to flow, liberating places where energy has been lying dormant to return us to the source of the divine flow. Our spine, when in alignment, allows the energy to soar throughout our vehicle.

THE "MUSCLE OF THE SOUL"

Let's continue on through our anatomical journey and meet some other pertinent muscles and bones to consider in this saga. The psoas muscle is key to this story of misalignment. It is so very important in the "management" of the movement of the legs in relationship to the pelvis and the spine. There are two psoas muscles, major and minor.

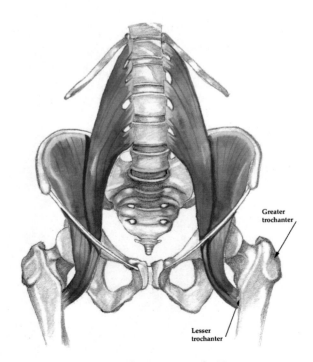

Greater trochanter

Lesser trochanter

The Psoas Placement on the Femur

The major attaches into the lesser trochanter of the femur bones (way up into the inner upper thigh), travels through the pelvic basin, continues behind the pelvic bones, and emerges out in the back body from each of the five lumbar vertebrae and T12 (the twelfth thoracic vertebra). It does not directly attach to the pelvic bowl; however, its influence on the pelvis is dramatic due to its relationship with the femur bones and ribcage. It passes over the ball and socket hip joint, connecting into the lesser trochanter, which directly affects the articulation and range of motion within the hip sockets and legs.

> *"These linings, wrappings, cables, and moorings are a continuous substance. Every single part of the body is connected to every other part by virtue of this network; every part of us is in its embrace."*
>
> **—Deane Juhan,**
> *Job's Body*

The minor originates at T12 and then grows into a thin tendon at the pelvic rim. To fully elongate the legs out of the pelvis, with the power moving through the earth, depends on the psoas. As the legs descend, the spinal muscles elongate in the opposite direction.

Liz Koch, author of *The Psoas Book,* proposes that our psoas, "literally embodies our deepest urge for survival, and more profoundly, our elemental desire to flourish."[29] The psoas serves to keep the body upright, extending the legs and keeping us moving. When the psoas is shortened, raveled, and tense, we cannot have the freedom of movement that allows us to feel that energetic surge of life force—we are literally imprisoned in our structure. Were we to know how to lengthen and release the tension in the psoas, how much more grounded would we be? How much more connected to the divine energy that we are, to source, and to the earth that we have such a great responsibility for?

Danielle Olsen, a yoga therapist, calls the psoas the "muscle of the soul."[30] Powerful words! This core-stabilizing muscle, a hip flexor, has the most important job of keeping us in motion, while simultaneously balanced, flexible, and upright. How can we live in the present moment when we are pulled consistently out of alignment? When our bodies are challenged and, perhaps, in pain, all we want to do is escape, and, if the pain is bad enough, take medication to eradicate it.

I must also mention the iliacus muscle, as it directly comes into play with the psoas. It fills the inner wall of the pelvic bones and together these two are called the iliopsoas complex. Together, they affect abdominal organ functioning, viscera, nerves, and the skeletal balance of the pelvic basin. As they share a common tendon, what occurs in one muscle will be reflected in the other.

As our alignment is so very challenged, with a pelvis that is thrust forward and tilted to one side, we cannot possibly make the best use of the psoas. It is literally pulled up and shortened like a raveled rubber band that is of a great thickness.

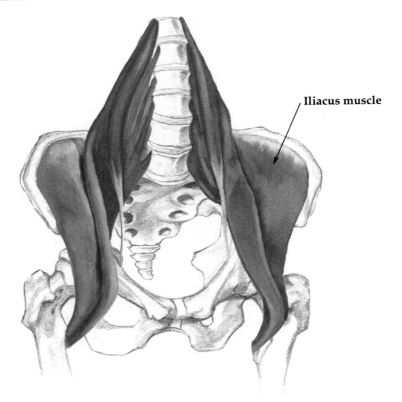

The Iliacus Musculature

How are we to extend the leg bones out of the pelvis, and allow the muscles to elongate naturally and freely? How can we extend the spine out of the pelvis with our muscles fighting to hold the structure up? Our very outer layer, the skin, reflects the distortion that is produced in the very core of our base, in our pelvic floor.

Remember looking into the mirror and seeing the wrinkles of your clothing creating pulls in the fabric? The design is different on each side of the body, muscles realigned in their own way due to the stretch of the fibers. The wrinkles you can see in your clothing indicate how the flesh beneath your clothing is also pulling.

With a base that is pulled up and contracted—often from our first entry into this body, perhaps due to fear, lack of safety, and not having a sense of belonging—this also produces enormous stress and tension in the pelvic floor, to the psoas muscle, and to all the muscles in our pelvis and low back, radiating throughout the whole structure.

FINDING YOUR CORE

I am sure you have heard the word "core" in your exercise classes over these last years. It has become a buzzword since Pilates arrived in the mainstream exercise world. What I have found so fascinating is that the understanding of where the core resides is quite mysterious. In the study of embryology and original movement, we learn that we are moving bodies that have gone through many designs to become the one we now are. We have hundreds of thousands of years of development and transformation and the seeds of this design lie within us.

> *"...the letting go of control, the letting go of self. This is surrender to the mystery of life."*
>
> **—Alan Lightman, American Physicist and Author**

What is so exciting about this for me, as I assist others in discovering stagnant places, is the realization that as moving beings, bodies that continue to evolve and heal, this place we call the "core" is shifting and changing. What does it mean to be "in tune," to be in alignment, to move with the grace of this magical design? And how do we find our core movement, our original movement?

Dona Holleman, a yoga teacher and author who I had the honor of practicing with many years ago in my B.K.S. Iyengar Yoga training, expressed this sentiment so beautifully when she spoke of "an innocent body." Remember the baby who squats effortlessly to the floor? In our beginnings, living in this amazing structure, we moved with freedom and abandon as we ran, skipped, and played, challenging ourselves and never really attending to how we could possibly do all this. Over time, "glitches" in the system appear—a fall, a repetitive tweak in the back, collapsed arches, stiffness in the mid-back that turns into an ache, a pain in the neck. These opportunities can shine a light on what might be a pattern worth investigating.

How would our lives be different had we had the understandings of structural alignment and a body which can rely on the bones to remain in anatomical balance? After all, it is the bones that should be dictating our structure, not the muscles that pull on them. As Holleman writes in her book *Centering Down,* "The muscles should not have any 'opinion,' they should not hold the bones in a way different from their structure."[31] Yet, throughout our lifetime, we have distorted muscle over and around bones causing misalignment and a structure that learns to demand that we move in distorted patterns resulting in greater havoc. When muscles adhere to the bone, they form quite strong opinions and take control of the structure in the best way they know how to carry it. "The bones, muscles and skin should 'fall apart'," she writes, "then the finer energy of the body is released and the body becomes innocent." What a beautiful way to express the majestic form in which we are embodied. It is not an easy form to stay aligned in; however, with awareness, it is one that we can reclaim.

"Your body will remember what your mind doesn't. Trust this."

—Anita, a client

For now, in the beginning of your investigation and discovery of your distortion, think about your core being located behind the pubic bone. Your abdominal muscles lie beneath there and begin there. We usually connect with the abdominals higher up, however, with a pelvis out of alignment we cannot access these deepest muscles. A pushed-forward pelvis wreaks havoc with all the attachments on the pelvis and of course into the legs. The femur bones are pulled out of alignment with the huge quadriceps muscles misaligning on them.

Remember the notion I introduced in the previous chapter of the "front body" and the "back body"? Now, imagine creating a conversation between them to create a healthy core. In order to elongate ourselves out of the sacrum, from behind the sacrum, we must have space. We must position the pelvis in an anatomically released manner as this structure is like a mannequin with muscle freely hanging off bone, allowing the bones to elongate, and support us, align us with the energy of the earth and connect us to source. The spine is the electrical conduit for the flow of energy; to untwist the holdings and free up the flow to every organ system is our intention.

THE FASCIA

Several years ago, I had the honor of hearing a presentation by Richard Schleip, PhD, long-time Rolfer and foremost fascia researcher. I was mesmerized listening to his description of the amazing connective tissue known as the fascia. This fibrous network, similar to a spider's web, is made of mostly collagen. It covers all the organs, nerves, arteries, veins, muscles, and bones. One continuous fabric, it literally holds the structure of the body intact. When the body is under stress of any kind, emotional as well as physical, micro-tears appear in the densely woven fabric of the fascia, and this organ-like structure begins to realign by pulling, torqueing, and twisting structures internally out of alignment.

This information is vital in understanding distortion and pain. In its normal unharmed state, the fabric of the fascia is supple, relaxed, and wavy. In stressful states, be it an injurious car accident, emotional stress, or any trauma, it loses its elasticity. Habitual poor posture and misalignment is also a stress, and the structure of the fascia, according to Schleip is compromised. As we age, this fibrous network becomes fibrotic (like scar tissue) and as it covers every organ, muscle, and bone, he writes, "We must think not only biochemically as we age, but biomechanically."[32]

This resonates with what I have observed in my work with people. The pressure put on the muscles, bones, and organs when the pelvis is out of alignment causes restriction of movement and most importantly, in the aging process, has the body "locked" into threatening positions. The fascia, the container that holds us together, is compromised.

WHAT IS CORRECT ALIGNMENT?

If you look at the image of "correct alignment," you can see the line drawn through the crown of the head, down the spine, through the pelvic floor, and into the earth. Angela Farmer, a world-renowned yoga teacher and one of B.

K. S. Iyengar's earliest students, used to speak of the area at the base of the buttocks as the "eye behind the thigh" and I have come to use this metaphorical image with all my students and clients. If you are old enough to remember the mannequins in the store windows that were never able to balance on two legs, you may also remember the steel rods that emanated from the base of the butt, from this place called the "eye." The "eye" is located just below the "sit bones" at the fleshy meeting of the buttocks and the thigh (sometimes called the "smile line"). In fact, we must never sit on the sit bones (the ischial tuberosities), those bony knobs that sometimes dig in to the floor if you ever find yourself there sitting cross-legged, such as in meditation or in a yoga class. With the perineum open all the way around we can sit in front of these spaces on the "eyes."

> *"Our muscles, encased and surrounded by fascia, can be perceived as the 'engines' responsible for producing the movement of our bony levers through space."*
>
> **—Irene Dowd**

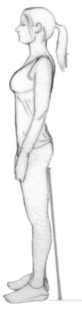

"The Eye Behind the Thigh"

When we stand, we must have that space in the top of the thigh and in the back body so that the sacrum can hang. Only then will muscle be able to soften over bone and free the bones from the musculature imprisoning us. The sacrum is extremely thick and aids in supporting and transmitting the weight of the body.

Let's focus our attention on some of the sacral muscles, which stretch from the sacrum to the spine of the hip bone (the ischium), and bring freedom of movement to the sacrum and low back and all the way up to the head. The piriformis muscle is also very important as it fans out from the sacrum to the upper thigh, where it attaches on the large trochanter of the upper thigh. As a result of this placement, it is able to externally rotate, abduct, extend and stabilize the hip joint. While this muscle and the psoas are not directly part of the pelvic floor array, we can begin to understand how they come into play with a pelvis out of alignment. The piriformis stretches diagonally to the sacrum and with other muscles, the obdurator externus and internus, serving to turn the leg outward. If this muscle is shortened, if one side of the piriformis is stretched tighter than the other, the sacrum is torqued.

The coccygeus muscle inserts on the lower sacrum and supports the pelvic cavity and is able to flex the sacrum. The iliacus also has fibers originating from the sacrum, and those attach to the lesser trochanter of the femur, allowing it to flex the thigh at the hips and stabilize the hip joint. Another muscle, the multifidus lumborum, which is the deepest muscle arising from the sacrum, helps stabilize the spine. And the erector spinae is essential in achieving extension and lateral bending of the head and the vertebral column.

I mention all of these not to confuse you or suggest you learn the intimate details of pelvic floor anatomy, but to show how many muscles are involved in our movement stories. The tweaks and torques deep in the floor of the pelvis create whole new patterns as we move this body over time.

We have been conditioned in exercise classes to harden muscle. Bones will never slide behind muscle that is literally glued together. With the awareness of fascia, now imagine the layering of distortion. As a child, we learned to walk and squat in perfect alignment. We can get back there. It is not hard to do, however, the neurology is a tough competitor for our awareness or the lack of it. Moving in set patterns for most of a lifetime, the brain, the neurology, firmly believes that *it* knows how to carry out the job of carrying the structure through the world. It certainly does, albeit in distortion and pain!

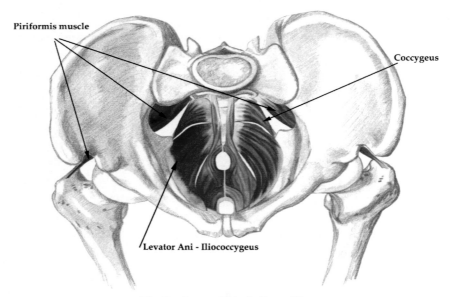

The Pirformis Muscle Front View

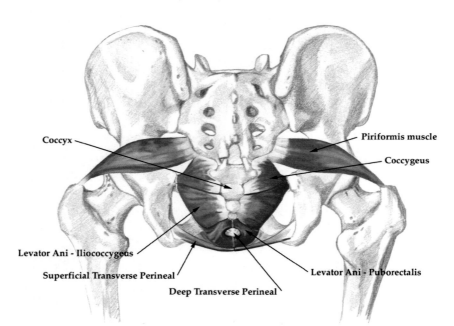

The Pirformis Muscle Back View

The real brain—the deeper intelligence—is in the cellular structure. As the cells of the muscle fiber begin to realign on bone with the new special awareness you are creating in your practice, millions and millions of cells inform each other and ultimately inform the brain. It takes longer for the brain to "get it" as we have been encased in these movement patterns for so many years. The good news is that when we free up the structure, the memories of where we began surge back in.

While I have shared a lot of information here, I do not intend for you to become an anatomy specialist. As I've already stated, my intention is for you to begin having light bulbs go off as to how your particular journey of pain might have evolved. It's all about *space* in the *base!* When we awaken and cultivate the knowledge and develop the tools, we change, we heal.

TOUCHING THE DIVINE, TRANSFORMING THE PELVIS

What other aspects of our divine being do we lose connection to as we shut down our energetic pathways? Sexual dysfunction is closely related to pelvic problems, and releasing the pelvis may open new pathways for our sexuality to express itself. This is what my dear friend, John Maxwell Taylor, author of *Eros Ascending,* has to say on sacred sexuality:

> What if an essential aspect of emerging from the embryonic state of dormant, unconsciousness, transformative potential in which humanity has existed for aeons, is propelled by an organic evolutionary impulse to give new birth to ourselves as a race? And suppose this process is somehow bound up with redefining our relationship to our sexuality? If we can let ourselves consider that our sexual impulses are, at their core, an expression of our innate divinity, then a new sense of responsibility may arise in regard to the way we approach the tremendous transformational power of conscious sexuality. By putting Eros and Psyche together, we can free ourselves to ascend from the depths of unconscious confusion about sex, and religion, and move towards clear spiritual and personal self-perception through the direct experience of ecstatic divine love. What sane person would not wish to embrace personally and support such an emergence collectively?[33]

We are indeed more than we could ever imagine. To open our structure, to return to receivership with a willingness to become more and belong more is a magical mystical journey. Given the tools, and the map of body awareness, we can unlock precious doorways to the divine life connection we have yearned for.

For further resources to support your inquiry, including videos, guided audio exercise, and more visit:

www.corebodywisdom.com

CHAPTER 4

THE MEMORY OF THE CELLS: HOW EMOTION AND BELIEF INFORM THE BODY

"The ground of your being is the pelvic floor, to drop down through your body and to rest there is to come home to yourself."

—Philip Shepherd, *New Self New World*

WE ARE THE architects, the designers of our structure. This thought arose, unexpectedly, as I was working with a longtime client. Together, we were journeying with meditative awareness into the recesses of the pelvic floor, discovering where the tributaries of energy were not flowing. My insight penetrated beyond muscle and bone and I began to recognize how the ways in which we have inhabited the body have created confusion and distortion at a cellular level.

Our cells have accommodated the body's distortion. As brilliant designers, we have created a story on this physical plane that mirrors the deeper patterns of our history—culturally, emotionally, and spiritually—and throughout hundreds of thousands of years of evolution. We arrived in this body with historical tomes of information preceding us, informing us, creating our beliefs, our map of awareness. As we have seen in the previous chapters, this information includes the previous forms through which we have evolved—our evolutionary predecessors, our human ancestors, our own embryonic stages. It includes the physical and emotional events of our own lifetime as well.

In some ways this can be quite soothing, and in other ways quite disconcerting. I am the product of a heritage that came way before I ever existed and yet informs my cellular awareness (or lack of awareness) every moment. This design that becomes *me* is indeed a mystery and yet one that I carry with me everywhere. And it produces information on a cellular level that keeps informing me. Unawake and unaware as to the presence of these ancient dormant patterns that are so much a part of my physical, emotional, and mental history, I might be perpetuating old scenarios and allowing them to still define me. This keeps me responding in old ways, crystallized in ancient stories, beliefs, and behavior patterns.

In this chapter, I want to take a closer look at how this information is carried, in our cells, and how it affects us. We may think that our physicality has become designed by how we have used this body, and that is true to some extent, as we have seen in the previous chapters. However, there is so much more input as to who we are becoming from the very moment of conception and even before. Since we have focused in some detail on the physical, anatomical level, I will now turn my attention to the less tangible but no less powerful material of our beliefs, emotions, and traumas.

"Health and disease are not built into the genes. They are built into our perception of our felt environment."
—Bruce Lipton

Over the past few decades, tremendous progress has been made in understanding the relationship between mind and matter and, specifically, between mind and body. We certainly have evolved our thinking as to how patterns emerge that lead to discomfort, tension, stress, and illness, and we now know that there are a variety of factors that come into play in "the creation of disease." Only some of these are physical.

To discuss the nature and behavior of matter and energy without considering environmental factors now seems to be a most outdated approach, although this is by no means embraced by all scientists (the old nature versus nurture conversation). Science has believed for some time that genetics are the primary controlling factor in the formation of disease, but it is now becoming apparent that this is too narrow a conclusion.

The newer science of epigenetics purports that the environment controls the fate of the cells. Hence, the environment controls biology. Genes are the blueprint that makes the parts of the body—the cells—but they do not control biology. Epigenetics brings to Western medicine a new understanding of the development of abnormalities in the cell structure and, ultimately, to the creation of disease. The field is still in its infancy, but what it tells us is that our genes are influenced by many more factors than scientists previously realized. In his book *The Biology of Belief,* developmental biologist Bruce Lipton writes:

…*Epigenetics*, which literally means "control above the genes," has completely upended our conventional understanding of genetic control. Epigenetics is the science of how environmental signals select, modify, and regulate gene activity. This new awareness reveals that our genes are constantly being remodeled in response to life experiences. Which again emphasizes that our perceptions of life shape our biology.[34]

The implications of this are profound. It means that we, as the "driver" of this physical vehicle, have a lot of input in shaping it—not just the muscles or the bones but the cells and the genes themselves. How do we shape them? Through life experiences and perceptions. In other words, we see our decisions, our behaviors, our feelings, our thoughts, our beliefs, and our attitudes reflected back to us in the vitality or the lack of vitality of our bodies.

From one perspective, this could sound harsh. "You mean my pain is my fault?" I've heard more than one person ask. It is not my intention to blame you for the physical form you find yourself in. Certainly, genetics play an important role too. For example, on a genetic level there are abnormalities that create specific responses or birth defects. But you play more of a role than you may realize. Much of it is happening subconsciously—it's not like you sat down and decided to create your disease or distortion. But bringing awareness to how your lifestyle and beliefs may influence the distortion in your cellular structure is important.

> "Inner alignment is the voluntary relation of a human being with a greater movement. Inner alignment is when I make myself available, when I deepen my listening and my awareness of the movement I am swimming in."
>
> **—Thomas Hübl,**
> **The Mystical Principles of**
> **Healing**

Specifically, I intend to shine a light on the patterns that have been formed in states of unawareness, and under acute conditions of stress. When our hormonal system is in a state of high alert and panic, we learn ways to "control" negative outcomes. At the time, we believe that these behavior patterns are protecting us. All the while, under the many layers of shadow, there lies our original decision to protect ourselves.

What I have learned personally and with the trust of those that come to me for guidance is that awakening consciousness connects us to the original movement of our life force, which is always there ready to inform us. How we have diverted this movement, for whatever reasons, has resulted in lack of movement, created tension and stress, and often provided the atmosphere for disease to evolve. So while you may not have consciously chosen illness and pain, you may well have been unconsciously choosing to be asleep to your patterns—patterns you have no idea you inherited. This is, perhaps, a more accurate and helpful way to think about decisions you might have made while unaware.

We must have enormous compassion for this journey we are on. Because the organism and the life force want to thrive, they will create an assortment of behaviors to do just that. There are so many stories embedded in the structure of the cells, and many of those stories are pushed away, discarded, and negated, and keep informing us in ways we are not awake to.

As we contemplate how we have protected ourselves from feeling our less-than-joyous experiences, and recognize the impact this has had, we can also find more courage to embody our joy. It's an extraordinarily empowering awakening. As Lipton says, "The new science of epigenetics (control above the genes) promises that every person on the planet has the opportunity to become who they really are, complete with unimaginable power and the ability to operate from, and go for, the highest possibilities, including healing our bodies and our culture and living in peace."[35]

BELIEFS CONTROL BIOLOGY

Lipton is one of my heroes. Let's take a closer look at his powerful insights. As a scientist, he was for some time misunderstood for his realization, "that a cell's life is controlled by the physical and energetic environment and *not* by its genes."[36] Lipton was convinced that it is a single cell's "awareness" of the environment, not its genes, that sets into motion the mechanisms of life.

Imagine the disturbance this created in the world of cell biology and beyond. His research at Stanford between 1987 and 1992, was a precursor to the field of epigenetics. Ultimately, he stopped teaching at the medical school because he could not support the belief that genes are the ultimate controllers. For this he received a lot of push back, for it ran counter to the established rhetoric of the scientific community. His research and understanding validates for me that our life stories—the circumstances we have been born into and the historical narratives that keep informing us—are a deeper response to an environment that we have not been even remotely aware of. Although unseen, it has determined the way we think, feel, react, (love, hate, judge), contract and expand. In short, our lives are based upon how we perceive and how others have taught us to perceive. Lipton calls this the "belief effect."[37] Our perceptions, accurate or inaccurate, equally effect our behavior and our bodies.

This holds for beliefs that are held in the muscle-fiber cells, which may limit movement and flow. As soon as we enter a body we become set, crystallized in patterns. As Lipton writes, "By definition, a structure whose molecules are arranged in a regular repeated pattern is defined as a crystal."[38] Not all crystals are alike, however. "We can be hard and resilient," he states, "or that crystalline organization can allow the membrane to alter its shape while maintaining its integrity and be fluid like a liquid crystal."[39] This idea of crystallization resonates with my own work. Crystallized energy is held within the cell structure that we so creatively designed when we did not feel safe, needed to protect ourselves, withdrew from negative stimuli, contracted, and pulled up out of our base, producing hardwired pathways that became habits.

Our behavior, on a cellular level, is controlled by how we have hardwired our beliefs. We wear the misperceptions of others: teachers, parents, friends; the many we cross paths with; and those that walked the earth for hundreds of thousands of years before we arrived. These programmed misperceptions in our subconscious mind— misperceptions that are not monitored because we are not awake to how they have been formed—will habitually engage us in inappropriate and limiting behaviors.

If you find it hard to accept that beliefs can be carried biologically, consider this example. In Argentina, a champion polo pony named Califa was cloned. While the ethics of this practice have been questioned, the experiment worked quite well. Their breeders believe that their horse clones are born with a type of shadowy memory inherited from their donor "parents." They told *Vanity Fair,* "From a very early age they know things that no one has ever taught them." These behaviors are stored not just in the brain "but encoded in every cell of the body." The breeders believe that when the adult horse is cloned, these "cellular memories" are copied along with the DNA." The champion Califa was a case in point. The original Califa had an intense fear of garden hoses, and his owner reports that its clone is equally terrified of them.[40]

"Through the conditioned learning process, neural pathways between eliciting stimuli and behavioral responses become hardwired to ensure a repetitive pattern,"[41] Lipton writes. "It is the job of the membrane in a single cell to be aware of the environment and set in motion an appropriate response to that environment."[42] The membrane, he says, is the cell's equivalent of the brain. It receives signals or messages. For example, stress comes to the membrane and the cell reacts according to what it knows, how it can survive. The cell is put on alert. What do I do now? How do I best react?

Hormones play a role here as well. Chinese medicine teaches that the hormones affected by trauma and stress cause us to enter a state of fight or flight—especially the adrenal gland, though all hormones are challenged by stress. Like energetic soldiers, hormones flood the internal field and the cell membrane is called into active duty, to stand guard, to protect in any way it knows how to. In this way, hormonal imbalance causes energetic dissonance.

Eventually, with all the possibilities and subconscious programming, the choices become automatic. What is known behavior? What was used before? It could have been something learned by our ancestors thousands of years ago or a behavior learned from a parent. Lipton explains that, informed by the cellular behavior pattern, these functions have been taken over by the specialized group of cells we call the nervous system.

Thanks to insights like these, the question of *how* we become *who* we become is not such a big mystery anymore. The awakening process in the formation of what I call our "Life Book" becomes more and more apparent as we witness our reactions and behaviors. These formations of our design need to be held tenderly as our heart becomes informed by our beginnings.

The energy that does not flow through open conduits creates distortion. It interferes with the ability to stay tuned to specific environmental signals. We have receptor proteins that monitor the internal landscape of the cell and other receptor proteins that extend from the cell's outer surface monitoring external signals. Information comes in from the environment and we also interpret what we perceive and project those interpretations onto the world around us. Bruce Lipton says that these receptors (integral membrane proteins, or IMPs) are the cell's sense organs, the equivalent of our eyes, ears, nose, and taste buds. These "nano-antennae" are tuned to specific environmental signals. He writes, "Cells possess a uniquely 'tuned' receptor protein for every environmental signal that needs to be read. The receptor-effector protein complex acts as a switch, translating environmental signals into cellular behavior."[43]

Is it becoming clearer how we become *formed*, how we become the mirrors of *in*formation, and how we are *in*formed and *out*formed? The role that energy plays in biological systems is vital, according to Lipton. Receptors can read energy fields. "Biological behavior can be controlled by invisible forces, including thought."[44] Once he understood how IMPs worked, he concluded that the cell's operations are primarily molded by its interaction with the environment, not by its genetic code. The cell must create an appropriate response to whatever environmental signals are presented. "When the electrical charge on the protein is altered, the protein changes shape"[45]; "… cytoskeletal proteins regulate the shape and the motility of cells."[46] Our very structure is altered and we are redesigned again and again by a series of external and internal reactions. We are the architects, the designers, building ourselves in reaction to the shifts and alterations.

The flow of energy that has been squelched and misdirected has profound effects—physically, emotionally, mentally, and spiritually. Our light has been dimmed and we have turned it down to manage the stories and the patterns that arise. Most important to consider is that we have created scenarios in body, mind, and spirit as a response to the enormous deluge of information fed into our system. On a cellular level, we are incredibly creative in our reactions to all trauma, including emotional trauma. When people awaken to the way muscles are distorted over bone, they begin to feel and see their habitual movement patterns in a new way. When they go deeper and feel the choices the structure responded and adapted to as a result of the stories that live many layers beneath the surface, cellular memory is activated. I believe memories are a living history within our cell structure that can be awakened, brought to the surface and when felt, heal. This makes it possible to redesign and transform distortions in the muscular patterns.

> *"There is no agony like bearing an untold story inside of you."*
>
> **—Maya Angelou**

The defenses that we create when we are very young protect us from experiencing the terror and the pain, distance us from the original wound of not feeling connected, cared for, and nourished. In order to survive, the child creates stories that allow denial of the original pain. The organism in its intelligence immediately recreates the energetic flow away from the original source of pain, the place the scar landed, and the cell structure receives this new information. Remember, the membrane surrounding the cell transmits messages into the cell. The enormous realization that there is danger, that one is not being cared for, is not safe, creates an intense vibration. Fear creates a panic, a shutting down, and the energetic movement of life's flow is rerouted. The cell constricts in response to the information, just as the body contracts and pulls back in response to a blow. The movement of energy along the cellular conduits is diverted with this new information. The messages literally reroute the energetic pathways and the original information, the original "blow," remains dormant until such a time when the being feels safe enough to allow its emergence. As we "wake up" to those memories, memories housed within each cell, the associated fear and pain emerges.

A PERSONAL JOURNEY

To illustrate how our responses to the challenges life presents become crystallized in the body, allow me to share a very personal story. My own experience of *lack* is truly what inspired me to seek just the opposite—an abundant life. Like many human beings, I grew up with the mantra, "There is not enough." My desire for more was okay to feel, but not likely to be received. This all added up, many years later, to the belief that "I am not enough, I do not deserve the fullness of my life, and I certainly do not know how to receive."

A family entrained by their culture and lineage to believe in lack produced generations that carried this subconscious belief. I experienced an intense level of depression amongst my family members, a feeling of not belonging, and an ingrained pattern of not having enough and not *being* enough. This showed up in the form of illness. Now I see the illness as providing a way out of having to be responsible for that which we have been gifted. It gives people something to focus on that will prevent them from experiencing the full joy and breath of life.

My mother, a deeply passionate woman, was fearful of her own strength and power. Although she was not conscious of it, it is clear to me when I look back that she decided that the family inheritance of heart disease was one to embrace completely. In fact, when I was the age of twelve, she told me that I, too would know about heart disease, as it is our family's destiny. "How strange," I remember thinking. I made a decision rather early on that I would discover the truth of who I was without the constraints of history.

How I knew to do this is a mystery, but what I was witnessing in my family unit was a choice to die, give up, and retreat. There wasn't much joy; just people channeling their energy into misery. The focus was always on what was not working, on lack. What happens to deeply passionate people who do not choose to express their gifts, who make the choice to be the victims of a story, who do not even seem to be aware they are in a story? In my family, they became violent, victimized, depressed, bitter, repressed, and always living in angst and fear. If I inherited anything I would say that fear was the biggest "gift."

As a child, I recall how my mother would release tension with long, mournful sighs. "Why are you sighing, Mommy?" I would ask.

"Oh, anxiety, you will know about that soon enough," was her reply.

Can you actually gift a lifetime of lack? Certainly we can gift a lifetime of belief and the action or inaction that adds up to recreating the same story. We can pass on the beliefs, the behaviors, and the traits that lead to recreating the same scenarios, be they physical, mental, or emotional.

During one of her heart bypass operations, my mother awakened in the intensive care unit enraged. "Did you see your father?" she barked. My sister and I, knowing full well that she held on to years of bitterness and anger, made the quick decision with eye contact over the bed to tell her that we hadn't, thinking this would be the path to less fury. Her response was dramatic and frightening. She was, of course, wired up, tubes supporting her weakening vitality. The machines began to wildly bleep and her heart rate, blood pressure, and vital signs all screamed panic.

> *"Emotions are the glue that holds the cells of the organism together."*
> **—Candace Pert**

At that moment, I reached for her hand and asked, "At what point does the anger no longer serve you?"

Her response: "You are damn right I am angry and I will be angry until the day I die!" The rage on her face, the arteries in her neck expanding with the emotional surge, was frightening to watch. At that moment I realized the choice she made.

"Mom," I said gently, "you aren't dying of heart disease, you are dying of a broken heart." Tears streaming down her face, she immediately cut off the floodgates and the hardness reappeared.

When I asked her why she stopped, she said, "It's a Pandora's Box, I cannot open it up."

"What will happen if you do?," I pressed.

"I will die," she declared.

It was so clear to me that she had it all wrong. "Oh, mom, you are closed off to your heart and have quickened death. You have chosen death, you have chosen fear."

At this moment, I think we both realized that she had gone as far in this lifetime as she chose to. And I realized so clearly that it is a choice, a choice not to feel the pain of the original wound. A choice to protect that which was so terrifying to acknowledge from the very beginning—how alone and vulnerable, unprotected she was. I say this not with judgment, but with the utmost compassion. I know that without the support to make other choices, she had no idea that she was recreating ancient patterns. Her belief that she was alone did not allow her the safety to seek support, since she never had that experience.

Years later, I had the honor of witnessing her death, her choice to die. I say "honor," because she has been my greatest teacher. The call came in the middle of the night, and my sister and I immediately made the arrangements to fly to her. There had been years of heart disease, pharmaceuticals, bypass operations. Now, as we entered the final chapter, she could not speak. When I asked her if this was her time to go, she nodded her head yes.

Years earlier I knew I had made a different decision. Just as she chose disease and death, I chose wellness. I chose responsibility for wholeness. She did indeed give me the greatest gift of my life, the knowledge that I can choose. After all, she chose, didn't she? The life force, that she so fearfully squelched, was informed by her lineage. Her cultural heritage produced the responses to her story. The need to protect her tender heart produced familial reactions that were hardwired in her cell structure. The cultural history of lack and survival imbued her cells and kept *in*forming and *re*forming the being that was my mom. This lack prevented her from wanting more and receiving more, and from challenging her concept of life. It is all she knew, and yet she also knew her strength and her will. And ultimately, she gifted me my ability to choose.

My decision to awaken created an intense, dramatic scenario. I did not have the tools to follow through on my desire to be different, act differently, and create my reality in a different manner. Remember, acting responsibly is having the tools with which to respond differently. Most importantly, I did not know that I had inherited the historic imbalances over many lifetimes. I would have to spend many years of peeling away my history of lack so I could truly honor my authentic self. But that process has given me the ability to help others unravel. I have chosen the body as my palate—the muscles, as they lie on the bones in all of their distortion, as an avenue to create balance. I know that this is one way in to the core of our being, and it is a magnificent one, as the muscles loosen their tight grip on the body and freedom emerges. We can stand in our bones and allow the body to take flight.

The way the body has learned to accommodate the stressful and challenging life journey must be considered—on the physical, mental, emotional, and spiritual planes. As we go through life, we set up the mechanisms to meander through the morass of the stories and come out as whole and functioning as possible. In the process, we bypass the shadows deep within. We are creating more story in our attempt to leave it all behind. I know that the behavior patterns I felt and witnessed had dramatic results in how I handled fear, anger, grief, shame, and the enormous lack of belonging.

Decisions I made many years ago to protect myself have born their effect on my physicality. I battled sciatica for many years. I also carried the effects of those early childhood experiences in my jaw—the violence in my home that had me withdraw within and clench in abject terror lived for years in my jaw. My teeth were eventually destroyed with the clenching and grinding. As I suffered through years of dental work, it was apparent that my response to the fear was to completely shut down my voice, clench my jaw. I had partnered with my biology, so to speak, to protect myself in the only way I then knew.

As I began to peel the layers off, the original terror began to seep out and *re*inform my cell structure. All these many years later, and most recently with my current dental experience, I could feel each tooth and area of my mouth in ways that had been hardened and protected. My dentist began to understand how post traumatic stress disorder, or PTSD, created my intense dental history. He gently supported me as I felt all the energy released from my jaw.

Interestingly, on an anatomical level, I learned that the upper palate in the jaw is the same dome shape as the perineal body. And not only did I clench my jaw in fear for my life, from the very beginning, I contracted in the floor of my pelvis, as a protection.

How else has my entire structure responded over the many years in all the nooks and crannies where I protected and held on, suffocating this precious energy body? I know that our bodies wear the stories of our history. I also know, however, that I did not genetically inherit the proclivity to heart disease. I do remember clearly making the decision not to accept that baton when my mother attempted to pass it to me.

PROPRIOCEPTION: WHO AM I REALLY?

Here is where I must introduce an important term: *proprioception*. It means "sense of self," and refers to the body's ability to sense itself and know how it is positioned in space. Because we have lived in a structure that is out of balance for perhaps a lifetime, the imbalance feels normal to us. Living in confused patterns doesn't feel confusing. It feels "right" even though there may be pain and tension in the musculature. The cells will keep informing us in the pattern we have created and will inform each other to keep the myth alive.

When the unraveling of muscle off bone takes place and movement is unleashed, our balance shifts, we are likely to feel confused and disoriented. We can only transform when there is enough space within the structure to begin to inform the neurology that a whole new configuration is emerging.

A major component of proprioception is "joint position sense." As far back as 1557, it was referred to by Italian scholar and physician Julius Caesar Scaliger as the "sense of locomotion." Later, in the 1800s, the rhetoric was of "muscle sense," which helped to develop the idea of physiologic feedback mechanisms. The discovery that commands are carried from the brain to the musculature and reports from the musculature are carried back to the brain was important in the study of movement and balance. In the 1900s, it was theorized that proprioceptors provided information about movement derived from muscular, tendon, and articular (joint) sources.

Over the years, research in the areas of balance, joint position, and movement have revealed that due to muscle memory, habituation, desensitization, and adaptation, the patterns that we create are "remembered" in the body as truth. I always tell my clients, as they are unraveling the constraints in the musculature starting in the pelvic floor, that the brain is the last to be informed! The change and knowledge is awakened within the muscle-fiber cells and they in turn will inform the neurology.

There have been many pioneers who have contributed to our understanding of the power of the energetic field. In 1895, D.D. Palmer, the founder of chiropractic, highlighted that the flow of energy through the nervous system is critical to health. The blockages, or the lack of energy flow through the spinal column due to the mechanics of the vertebral column, provide critical information. Palmer developed skills to assess and "tune" the flow of information by adjusting the bones in the vertebral column to release tension and allow better energy flow. Cranial sacral therapy releases the "kinks" in the garden hose of the spinal cord to unleash this energetic flow. In more recent years, Donald Epstein, who was once a traditional chiropractor, found that by focusing on specific "gateways" along the spine, energy could not only be released but lifetime stories held in the nervous system can be released. He developed Network Chiropractic (also known as Network Spinal Analysis). All of these approaches show us that undoing the tension provides the road back to our source of light and our destiny.

Philip Beach, the osteopath, acupuncturist, and embryologist I introduced in chapter two, uses the concept of "tune," which he defines as "the harmonious interaction of thousands of named anatomical structures."[47] His "archetypal postures" are designed to develop "tune" in the musculoskeletal system, allowing the structure to bring freedom back into movement patterns. He describes this as "the re-tuning of our musculoskeletal system back to deeply embedded morphological norms."[48] For Beach, hundreds of muscles and joints relating with as little friction and dissonance is "biomechanical tune" that will yield a structure moving in freedom with less demand on that structure. Take the stress off the body and the body is free to bend and move with ease.

"The songs of our ancestors are also the songs of our children."

—Philip Carr-Gomm, Archdruid of Sussex

The more the body releases stress from years of holding on and fighting musculature, the more highly attuned we can become as we open the pathways to more energy and more light flowing through the core, from divine consciousness, through the spine and into the base. When there are frozen areas, patterns that have become habitual, limit our movement. These patterns, be they physical or behavioral, are addictive and hard to change. They keep the structure imprisoned in the past. Until we awaken to our patterns, we will keep recreating more tension and more stress. Often, that awakening process arises when we are in pain.

The frozen crystallized patterns embedded in the cell structure are unleashed and the free flow of energy feeds the system all the way down into the base, or the pelvic floor. This freedom allows an attunement process to take place, a connection that allows for the flow of all possibility. Free to *be* the destiny we came here to manifest, our physicality radiates the light we are. Isn't that what we all deeply want? To take the constraints off the structure, and be our soul's greatest advocate, living in divine presence?

ANOTHER STORY OF TRAUMA AND HEALING

Emotional traumas are "worn" like clothing that no longer fits, yet often we are attached to these garments and refuse to outgrow them. Like our old patterns, they have provided safety. My client Julia had quite an intense story of abuse. Even though she had done a lot of psychological work, which had been deep and healing, her physicality continued to haunt her in painful ways. The story was living deep in her tissues and in the cells of her musculature. She had unknowingly "arranged" her structure to cope with the trauma, creating further and deeper pain. Remember, we are the designers and the architects, and we find creative ways to deal with the intensity of stress and tension because it serves us to do so. It is necessary, for our survival, until the moments of truth seep out into the light of day and there arises another opportunity to choose again.

Julia was ready for such an opportunity when we first met, at a class I was teaching on structural realignment integration at a local yoga studio. Her distortions were very apparent, and she herself was quite well informed about her own physical issues. Her description of where the blockages were that led up into her jaw on one side were accurate. She had studied anatomy as part of her professional career so she already knew a lot. When we started to work privately, it became clear to me where in her base she had "pulled up," contracted, and sucked in her energy field. We could follow the shut-down conduits and as the shifts started to shake her system up, we could trace the closing off of the channels from her base at the perineum, through her pelvis, all the way up her spine, into her neck, jaw, and head.

Years ago, as a child, Julia told me, she manifested her rage in her jaw. Like me, she was unable to speak her truth early on and this was the physical form her protection took. This set up the physical map she clothed herself in, not knowing that she was setting the stage for the physical life play that she was to embody. In her case, as in so many sad stories, the root trauma was sexual abuse. When children fall prey to this abuse, they are unable to be their own advocates. The fact that her abuser was a member of her own family is also not uncommon. Other family members were also abused, and others did not speak up in defense of the children they knew were in jeopardy. All of this was terrifying for the young one. There was no one to help, to go to, for the family was clearly in collusion with the story as were others in the community where she grew up. And no one would have believed this was going on, in a community that was so family oriented and child centered. Julia's self-protection was so profound that for years she had no memory of the abuse she had suffered. All she was aware of was the pain in her jaw that at times had her feeling paralyzed.

"It is not our genes but our beliefs that control our lives."
—Bruce Lipton

Years later, accomplished in her field, married, and having raised two successful children, the pain started to become more and more profound and the memories started to seep forth. Her awakening, along with the returning memories, and the energy they unleashed were all terrifying, like a tsunami about to break on the shore. She sought out the help of professionals and body therapists, breathwork modalities; she was desperate for anything that would awaken her to what she had experienced.

Julia was fortunate to have as her life-mate a husband who was willing to be the ballast in all ways that he could as she unraveled the depth of her pain. She pursued her true identity—an identity that had become layered over with the story that she "wore" and protected all the years until her fiftieth birthday—by confronting other family members, who, as it turned out, were unwilling to bring those memories to the surface.

Julia's reactions and compensations to her life, embedded with shame, guilt, and rage created the map, the design of the structure she inhabits, just as it does for all of us, even those of us with stories that are far less intense. Now in her seventies, she is still unraveling the dysfunction in her neck and jaw. She is still as committed as ever to releasing the energy that she closed off to protect herself. As her energy has gradually unleashed, over the years she found that the deep rivers flowing through her introduced her to the amazing energy- and light-worker she herself is, and she allows this energy to be the source for others' healing too as it flows through her.

Freedom is something that needs to be reclaimed. The sense of belonging that initially becomes us is initiated in our base. That is the source of our beginning. When we have to protect ourselves early on, we contract the base and close off to the endless possibilities that could become our reality. We do not want more, because there is not enough space to grow in to. We are starved and create our life stories despite those things that we may not want to have *in*form us. Remember, we are light energy and light carries information. I experience myself as "light in formation," always becoming more of my true essence. We continue to become the update of our being as we open to the potential and possibility we are.

I find it amazing to contemplate how the energy and power located in our base, when freed up, can heal on so many levels. Ultimately, the way we inhabit our bodies has repercussions not only physically, as aches, pains, and distortions carry us further away from balance, but the deeper effects on the energetic system. What came first? Did traumas that we came into this life bearing, create the physical story as the flow of light from source became dimmed? Did physical traumas via accidents and/or from abuse cause the body to distort in fear and protection? Did we become the direct descendant in our physicality of the parents whose energy we were born into and grew up with? All of these play a role in *in*forming us. Bruce Lipton writes, "It is not our genes but our beliefs that control our lives."[49] Living in love makes our cells respond one way, living in fear another. The patterns we live with and through depend on which choice we make.

For further resources to support your inquiry, including videos, guided audio exercise, and more visit:

www.corebodywisdom.com

CHAPTER 5

THE SACRED JOURNEY: HOW SPIRIT BECAME YOU

"If anything is sacred, the human body is sacred."
—Walt Whitman

WHO ARE YOU? As we have seen in these past few chapters, you are made up not just of physical matter but of layer upon layer of story, history, and accumulated experience. As we peel back the layers and unravel the distortions, we come into contact with our essence. In this chapter, I want to focus on that deepest level of who we are, before we became embodied beings.

Looking into the eyes of a newborn, into pure radiating light, there is no doubt of our inherent connection to divine source. At these moments, witnessing pure creation and creativity, can we even question the source of our beginnings? Can we question the collaboration that creates? Yet we do question, doubt, and separate from the river of intelligence that informs us.

When and why we disconnected is a whole other conversation, and one that is vital to engage in. Why would we disconnect? What are we disconnecting from? Source? Love? Light? How free are we in this structure and how intimate are we with the energetic flow of the river that informs us and asks us to receive this light in formation? Are we collaborators with our destiny or have we turned ourselves so deeply *away* that we fear feeling what is behind the doors and windows of our hardened places?

Remember, the goal here is to bring you back into a state of wholeness, coherence, congruence, and freedom. That also means a state of collaboration and alignment with the original divine energy that became you. Many of us only begin seeking this kind of wholeness when we are in crisis—a time when we tend to feel so separate from a greater force, and hence, separate from ourselves. Our separation from this energetic light leaves us in doubt that we are already connected and aligned with greater wisdom and knowledge. Therefore, we tend to look outside of ourselves for answers, when in fact, the answers we seek are already present and accounted for in our partnership with divine creative knowledge and wisdom. The path to healing, then, involves looking inside—rebuilding our connection with the deepest essence of who we are in relation to others.

To become disconnected from the soul river that informs us is terrifying for the organism and can be the source of great fear and anger. How are we fed? How do we receive nourishment? How do we live, unaware, in this physical divine home, slowly suffocating and yet yearn to be free? To be *re*minded moment by moment is an awakening path that allows us to not get caught in the web of the habitual, of the addictive. Yet, reconnecting can also evoke more fear as the barriers erected no longer serve and we are invited to fill empty spaces with more of the original truth that we protected ourselves from.

We live in a time when science and spirituality have begun to come together, weaving the fabric of our essence into a pattern that we are beginning to understand, and welcome. We *are* transforming, *re*forming, being redesigned as we move in to and with the flow of the evolutionary river. We have remained lying dormant in a fear-based global culture for so long, wearing the scars of our battles as we travel through energetic fields of lack, dependent on the medical industry (and religious hierarchy) to inform us when our system gets jammed and misaligned. We have given away our responsibility to others hoping that all will be revealed and we will make it through intact and maybe even happy.

SO MANY QUESTIONS

When you direct your attention to the deepest levels of your being, you may encounter more questions than answers. I invite you to become comfortable in this space of unknowing, of curiosity. Thomas Hübl says, "By staying with the questions, listening for the essential chi (energy) that is wanting to move, we become a walking answer."[50] This brings to mind the medieval book *The Cloud of Unknowing,* written by an anonymous mystic, who says that the answers can only be revealed through love, the love of the divine. We are that love.

Here are some of the questions we will "stay with" in these pages. What does awakened consciousness have to do with the perineum? What does our spirituality have to do with physical structure? How are we the design that Spirit intended us to become? How do we live in this home of the soul, clean out the cobwebs of beliefs, attitudes, and perceptions so we can *be* the reflection of the original movement that is divinely us? Why did we incarnate into this structure? What is our destined path that we are here to awaken to? How come it takes us so long to slough off the bonds of misperception and become the divine truth we are?

In my study of anatomy, I never doubted that the pelvic floor and specifically the site of the perineum, was the source of our anatomical dysfunction, leading to a whole array of possible worrisome and painful outcomes. Years of unraveling my own distortion and challenging physical stories brought me into my base and ultimately deeper into my perineum. Years of observing and working with bodies confirmed these connections. Following the distorted rivers of muscle fibers led me to feeling, seeing, and connecting these incongruent tributaries with the lack of energy flow. This allowed me to make the deeper connections as to the source of dysfunction.

Developing the tools to support unwinding these stories of distortion to the source of our beginnings had the light bulbs flashing for me. I made the connection between the distortions in our physical bodies and the energetic divine light that is our essence. Remember, as discussed in chapter 1, the perineum is the point of your origin—the original cells that became you. Therefore, it is also the site at which consciousness entered the physical body, the spring from which the divine river of energy that informs you burst forth.

> *"Consciousness is intrinsic; woven into the fabric of the universe."*
>
> **—Dr. Stuart Hameroff, M.D., Anesthesiologist**

Energy that is dammed, that is prevented from moving, has us ever more imprisoned in this physical structure. How to unleash energy that has been channeled and funneled through conduits that we are not even aware of due to so many physical, mental, and emotional stories? We keep ourselves so far away from the original flow of our divine river. We walk through life disconnected and fearful of connection.

The practice of yoga teaches us to awaken the channels at the base of the spine to receive light, energy, movement. The nerves that emanate from the base of the spinal cord—the "seat of knowledge," as the ancient scriptures call it—feed every organ in the body. But if this garden hose, as my friend de-

scribed it, is twisted in a variety of places along the pathways, can we receive
the flow of the cerebral spinal fluid, can we receive the light energy along the
conduits? Without movement, can we fully become that which we are here
for? How have the twists and torques, the misalignments, prevented the energy, the flow, from informing our vessel?

The more deeply I have connected to the energetic essence of who I am
and who we all are, the more profound this work has become. The purpose
of unraveling distortion in the muscle fibers is not only to free people from
physical pain, but to awaken and enliven the pathways that will allow people
to reclaim their energetic light. In so doing, they are empowered to enter the
field of evolutionary consciousness and play the part that they were meant to
play in the divine dance of creation.

SCIENCE AND SPIRITUALITY

Let's take a closer look at what science and spirituality teach us about who we
are. Typically, these two fields have been far apart, but today, they are con-
verging in exciting ways. Dr. Bruce Lipton was asked in an interview where
science and spirituality intersect, and he replied: "Quantum physics."[51]

I have neither the space nor the expertise to do justice to the topic of
quantum physics in this brief chapter, but what I find to be particularly important is the way in which it confirms the insights of the mystics with re-
gard to the existence of Spirit. Mystics, for millennia, have talked about the
invisible force that connects us. In fact, it might be one of the few things
all the religions agree on—that we are all connected to an unseen energetic
source. As spiritual teacher Eckhart Tolle, author of *The Power of Now*, writes,
"Underneath your outer form, you are connected with something so vast, so
immeasurable and sacred, that it cannot be conceived or spoken of—yet I am
speaking of it now. I am speaking of it not to give you something to believe
in but to show you how you can know it yourself."[52]

It is only recently that science has begun to acknowledge the existence of
this invisible "field" that shapes and influences matter. Science writer Lynn
McTaggart explains, "Human beings and all living things are a coalescence
of energy in a field of energy connected to every other living thing in the
world. This pulsating energy field is the central engine of our being and our
consciousness."[53]

What that means is that we are not really made of matter, we are made of energy. Albert Einstein recognized this when he said that, "mass and energy are both but different manifestations of the same thing."[54] And quantum physics essentially reveals that what we used to think of as the building blocks of reality, atoms, are in fact particles held together by the vibrating force of energy. Einstein put it this way: "The Field is the sole governing agency of the particle."[55] Quantum theory tells us that the observer—human consciousness—plays a role in "coalescing" these vibrating particles into what appears as solid matter.

This means that whatever reality we create is, in some sense, of our own design. The stories that we travel through—physical, emotional, or mental—*in*form, and *trans*form our being, as we bump into all the beliefs of the culture and the family lineage we are embedded in. To enter this human form with all that we inherit at the moment of conception is a journey that takes us from the most enlightened realm of pure divine energy into a "crystallized" structure that is contained and kept imprisoned in form. Our journey is to awaken to the light we are sourced from.

SPIRITUAL ANATOMY

Can we separate our individual experience from all that came before? Can we separate our bodies from the divine field of energy that influences everything?

Light is energy and we are sourced from this energetic explosion. We are light in formation, *in*formed by light; our awakened consciousness is energy in action. The place of our embodiment, the perineum, is the area also known as the root chakra. It is here that we experience our first awareness of being welcomed into this world, as everything that transpires between our parents is received and experienced in us, the new arrival. It is here that we experience safety or the lack of safety. As we entered through the karmic field—through thousands and thousands of years of collective history and collective trauma, decisions made and behaviors created—all of this is embedded in our cellular memory.

> *"Cells are sentient beings. We are the manifestation of our cells. Each of us is a cell in the body of a superorganism, in the body of humanity."*
>
> **—Bruce Lipton**

How connected are we to our energetic origins? How stuck, contracted, and withdrawn are we physically, emotionally, mentally? Are we just consumers of energy or are we creating a feedback loop where we are sharing energy?

We have the potential to live as awakened energy generators, curious and creative. To be grounded, we must have a free and awakened base, for this is when energy can flow, allowing inspiration and manifestation of our most creative ideas and aspirations to begin to *in*form *us,* to awaken us to our destiny. How will I fulfill this lifetime contract in which I partnered with the Divine? The base of our structural home, the perineum, is directly related to the light that enters through the crown at the top of the skull. This sacred energy housed within the light, which originally downloaded us into the body, is available to be accessed every moment. It is our connection to soul and beyond. To manifest our potential, we must have a physical structure that is open and free to receive. The correct anatomical alignment of the pelvis in relation to the legs and the upper torso, including the head, provides the freedom needed to access the light. Like a river with logjams of boulders and tree trunks our flow of energy has reduced movement due to the distortions of muscles pulling over and around bones.

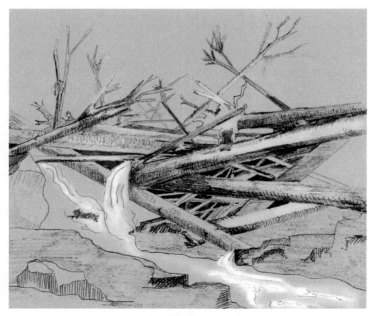

The Flow Impeded

Our security, stability, safety, and finding a "good home" within ourselves depends on our ability to ground ourselves. To be inspired, potent manifestors, creators, we must be grounded. The root chakra, when open and receptive, reconnects us to the source of light above the crown, which is connected to soul energy and to the very reason why we are here.

Personally, I spent most of my life not feeling grounded at all. I never felt that I truly belonged to any land that I lived on, not even the city of my birth. I could not find a place of comfort and safety. I have lived and participated in many communities, and even held leadership roles; however, I would never have said, "This is my place, the land where I feel at home. This is the place I want to make my permanent home." The home I grew up in was never a safe refuge. It was only when I landed in my base, remembering and releasing trauma, that I could come home in my own body and connect with all that came before. It was only then that I felt like I truly belonged to me. In belonging so deeply, I find myself wanting and willing to create roots, real roots, in body and in land, and as a deeper part of a transformational story in which I can play my part in bringing in the future.

CREATING HEAVEN ON EARTH

I hope you are now beginning to physically understand your connection to the greater wave of change—to see your own physical, emotional, and spiritual realignment as a critically important link to higher evolutionary consciousness and the transformation of our culture.

I was never a religious person, however, as a spirit awakening I am now more connected to the phrase "heaven on Earth" than I have ever been. I believe that awakening to our source, our divine essence, is what empowers us to play our part in transforming the world and the culture in which we live. In this sense, we bring divinity into the physical world—flowing through our own bodies and minds and informing the relationships we forge and the societies we create. This is also where we can talk about "evolution" in a new way—informed by our spiritual nature, we evolve ourselves, our consciousness, and our societies to be reflections of awakened divinity. We are evolution.

Professor Brian Goodwin, a Canadian biologist and philosopher, articulated a powerful vision for the coming together of science and spirituality.

He called on humanity to put nature and culture back together again, seeing ourselves not as observers and users of nature but as participants in nature. "The Great Work," he wrote in his last book, "the Magnum Opus in which we are now inexorably engaged, is a cultural transformation that will either carry us into a new age on earth or will result in our disappearance from the planet. The choice is in our hands. I am optimistic that we can go through the transition as an expression of the continually creative emergence of organic form that is the essence of the living process in which we participate."[56]

I see this vision of a "great work" coming up in many conversations today, where people's attention is moving from a focus on personal achievement and even personal spiritual growth to a focus on collective awakening and evolution. This shift from the "I" state of being to the "we" is at the core of our spiritual journey today. We are evolving as we acknowledge how deeply embedded we are in collective dynamics. We are moving from a personal need to consume more resources, even to consume spirituality and have it *inf*orm me, to a more collective awakening of sharing resources, relying and caring for each other and the planet on which we reside. Awakening to collective fields of consciousness, we are creating a new evolutionary stage, a new being.

"*There is a crack, a crack in everything, that is how the light gets in.*"
—**Leonard Cohen**

David Abram, a cultural ecologist, has written an exquisite book, *The Spell of the Sensuous*, in which he takes the reader on a journey to experience that all life forms are connected. He unfolds the mysterious relationship between science and mysticism. He challenges our habitual perceptions and encourages us to reorder our world within to receive a larger experience of what it means to be alive and embodied. Where we came from and how we *be*came who we are now is profoundly critical to understanding our human nature and our place in this ever-evolving journey we are part of.

When we awaken to the possibilities that life offers us at this point in our history we are called upon to be much more proactive and collaborative in the creation and awakening of our life pathways. As streams of energy are unleashed, decisions made in the past (from the need to protect) come to light, we now can integrate the past. This movement into the stream of life allows us to make new decisions with so much more information available, choosing a life in alignment. With alignment, light informs us more and more. And more light means more movement.

Every cell in our body is informed by this awakened consciousness—it informs our being and creates our path. What an astounding suggestion! And yet here we are, embodying the light. We all have moments when we recognize our essential nature, when we are completely amazed by astounding reflections of divine and awe-inspiring beauty. These moments have our hearts singing new energetic tones that resonate throughout the brain, throughout the spine, and awaken every nerve ending, connecting us to Source.

At many other moments, however, we are disconnected, confused, and unaware. The pathways energetically and physically receive less movement and less enlightened information. Our physical structure tries its best to house the reason we chose to be here in physical form this time, and cannot access all it needs to support us. Our physical structure collapses in response to our leaving our original design. It feels to me when I go away from the source of my beginning, from the divine knowing that is me, the body is weeping for losing connection. There is no one to care for me, as I have disappeared. The pain in my body is a much bigger story than the physical tale I told myself for so very long. This is why I call the journey "spiritual anatomy."

CONSCIOUSNESS NEVER DIES

Many of us believe that when we die, our consciousness dies with the physical body. But mystics both ancient and modern tell us that this is not true. The death of consciousness simply does not exist. It only arises as a belief because people identify themselves with their bodies. When we identify solely with the body, we subscribe to the belief that the body is going to perish, sooner or later, and then our consciousness will disappear as well. If we embody consciousness and live as generators of energy, does consciousness die when the body dies?

If the body receives consciousness in the same way that a cable box receives satellite signals, then of course consciousness does not end at the death of the physical vehicle. In fact, consciousness exists outside of constraints of time and space. It is able to be anywhere: in the human body and outside of it. In other words, it is non-local, it resides everywhere universally. Dr. Robert Lanza, M.D., a scientist that *Time* magazine cited as "100 of the most influential people in the world in 2014" is an expert in regenerative medicine and "the standard-bearer for stem cell research," according to *Fortune* magazine.

"Life and consciousness are absolutely fundamental to our understanding of the Universe,"[57] he writes, and he goes on to propose that "life creates the Universe, not the other way around."[58] Intelligence, this implies, existed prior to matter.

It is consciousness, intelligence downloaded into our human form, that comes with a wealth of energetic information that I believe keeps informing us.

Why do I feel that this is relevant to our discussion on becoming a fully embodied human being? Because if consciousness, as energy, always exists, then as an awakened conscious human we have access to so much more information than we can possibly imagine. If the vehicle we are driving is congested, distorted, or misaligned, how can we be the receivers of what Thomas Hübl calls Divine FM? Is our body attuned to be able to listen? What information are we listening to? We are not separate from all of the intelligence that is the universe. It seems to me that as sacred beings we have been gifted far more than we are ever aware of. When the light is turned on, when we access the energetic flow of the divine river, we *be*come that which our original contract intended us to be. Thus, we *be*long to a far greater intelligence. The freedom that we are and the intimacy that is exponentially our birthright becomes a reality.

For further resources to support your inquiry, including videos, guided audio exercise, and more visit:

www.corebodywisdom.com

CHAPTER 6

REMEMBERING THE BODY: HOW TO REACTIVATE YOUR INNER WISDOM

"When you set an intention, the whole universe changes."
—Markus Hirzig

LET'S LOOK AT where we have journeyed thus far in preparation to create a map by which to physically undo distortions that are causing disruptions and symptomology in the physical structure. It can be daunting to consider that this form we inhabit has been designed and shaped with information downloaded through thousands of years. By jumping over places that challenged and frightened us in the past, we were also prevented from receiving important information as we cringed and withdrew from ourselves.

In taking such detours, covering up those parts that were traumatized, where does that energy become stored and how have we become misshapen as a result? We now see how energy stored and hidden has an effect not only on our emotional and mental states but also on our physical states. What does this unraveling look and feel like? How can you take the body's story apart and reawaken the cell structure to welcome new possibilities? How can you create the room, the space, the freedom, to enliven—to not just live but to thrive in joy.

This journey we are on together—this journey to *be*coming the being we are meant to be and *be*longing to eons of fabric that preceded us—has included some detours along the path that has disengaged us from Source. We have become disenfranchised from our innate awareness of our connection to the light and the energy of higher consciousness that is our very essence. I know, deep in my own exquisite being, that I dimmed the light, diminishing myself in my own presence. Each of us has willingly and not so willingly separated from the ancient wisdom that is our birthright and informs every cell of our being.

This *we*, the collective *we*, has evolved through generations of story, creating contractions that deepen the wrinkles of fear, anger, sadness, and shame. These energetic confusions, wound-up crystallized spirals, have us redesigning our physicality in ways that oftentimes we hardly recognize ourselves. How long we have searched for the answers to questions that are in the fabric of our rich heritage? Love lives in the cell structure of our original design. Love is the fabric that feeds us. Dimming the light of love effects our emotional and mental states and the latter informs our physicality, leaving us caught in a web that is often convoluted and separates us even further from our inner wisdom. This body holds all the stories, all the decisions, like an encyclopedic memoir written in the fabric of the cells.

> *"We all compose the atmosphere of the human experience."*
> —**Thomas Hübl**

What does it mean to belong? What do we belong to? So much of our global population views "the other" or in Thomas Hübl's lexicon "the stranger" as different and dangerous. We are attempting, although unsuccessfully, to live in protected bubbles separated from what has us so terrified: each other. Ironically, this fear has kept us separated from ourselves, has resulted in our energy being sequestered in the crevices of protection. We learned this through thousands of years of downloaded information creating the design we now are. We become the stranger to ourselves as we close off from the love and light that we are.

The human organism, like all life forms, suffocates from the disconnection from higher frequencies. The love that we are by design has been leeched out of the cell structure, leaving us bereft, scared, and protected, as well as fearful of what lies beyond. The light we divinely embody, the inspiration that becomes the human form we live through, is our greatest teacher. The journey to feel love divinely must take us back to the beginning, unwinding with a depth of compassion that has us bowing down as we journey forward into truth. No longer strangers to ourselves, we meet the world with the shades drawn up!

Stephen Busby, whose work focuses on healing through higher consciousness, speaks of exposing ourselves to higher frequencies and how these frequencies allow the organism to vibrate and respond differently. "The whole organism begins to shift into the potential for a different alignment; an alignment *with* the higher frequencies,"[59] he says. We have the potential to source information that expands the bandwidth from which our creativity flows. Energies can flow through the layers of crystallized structure and change the patterns and the design. "Coming into alignment," he proposes, "is the next best version of ourselves."[60]

Open and awake, we continue to *become* our truth, the one that entered this energetic field and was perhaps taken astray through life incidents, thoughts, and beliefs. We experience belonging to a far greater field and do not feel the separation that might have been so necessary for our protection earlier in life. Channels are open for information to be downloaded through conduits that were previously congested and the body/mind organism tunes in, becomes attuned, and plays songs with new resonance and passion. New songs are created that never were played before as we evolve into a new being.

Evolution does not cease; we might slow it down, and we might also join the rivers that came before and bring forth those that are streaming in as we evolve into a new awareness, a new body. What courage it takes to bring forth the next best version of ourselves, to evolve, transform, and step into a brand-new alignment never before experienced. Physical alignment opens pathways to align ourselves with far greater fields of expanded consciousness.

AWAKENING TAKES PLACE IN THE MOST AMAZING PLACES

It was the middle of the night and the light of the full moon cascaded into Machu Picchu, the sanctuary created by Incan Empire. The travel group I was with entered at midnight, with the shaman guiding us through history, to rooms in which rituals were once performed that connected the inhabitants of this most sacred citadel to their ancestors, to the source of their beginning. Rooms with crevices carved into the walls where the Inca would enter and pass through the veils of illusion, not only into the past but into the future. During the day, the majesty of this structure, an architectural wonder surrounded by mountains and perched high above sea level, kept its inhabitants in a protected, secure environment. At night, the separation between the veils seems much thinner, and the shadows create the stage for information to stream in. In the dark my edges were less defined, my attachments to what I think I "know" less available. My solar plexus quivered with anticipation.

My fellow travelers and I had been together for several years studying the ways of the Peruvian Indigenous Peoples, exploring healing in the light body. We journeyed deep into rituals honoring Pachamama, or Mother Earth, guided into the realms of the Quechua Medicine People, an indigenous culture informed by the light and the stars and those that came before them.

While the moonlight bathed the city, I took my turn and stepped up into the hollow carved into the wall, where a people much smaller than I fit easily, as if cradled by the stone. I could feel the many that had preceded me and welcomed me. Friends and shamans drummed, rattled, and sang, bringing me into a field of consciousness imbued with sanctity for life connected to Divinity, gods with human attributes. The Quechua knew that without the love, honor, and respect for the land and the belief that supernatural forces govern everyday events, they could not survive. This connection was everything that kept them tethered to the land, Mother Earth, Pachamama. Their belief in these forces governing the weather and illness led them to make offerings in honor to the land that feeds them. The community depended on such honor, depended on receiving all that came before them to initiate them into the present and guide them into the future.

"...Cells communicate with each other by simply touching; all this goes on continually, without ever a personal word from us. The arrangement is that of an ecosystem."

—Lewis Thomas, *The Lives of a Cell*

My body merged into the stone, becoming more and more fluid, my edges of awareness expanding into cold stone that became permeable and warm as I sank in, deep. It was a cold night and yet the warmth that welcomed me melted the strain, the pressure keeping my structure intact. However, I was no longer "intact" as I merged into a presence I no longer had words to express. The stories I came with, my personal ones and all those that came before, no longer informed me and yet I brought all of myself through the veil. These veils parted and my consciousness reenergized—awakened me to information I could not even attempt to express. The indigenous people of this sacred land informed me, informed my consciousness, my cell structure, and carved new pathways for the light to stream in. Was I experiencing what is termed *awakened consciousness?*

In previous years, journeying through the veils of illusion and awakening pathways that I never knew nor felt, I had come to understand how my perceptions became deep defenses on all planes, physically, emotionally, and mentally, how I locked in patterns that kept me asleep and safe in distortion. Physical pain cannot be considered separate and treated without the unraveling on all planes of existence. Through profound journeys with the Qechua medicine shamans in Peru and my guides in the United States, I felt the fabric of my being redesigned—perception, beliefs, and habitual patterns released. I began to awaken to an energy that I had kept so deeply protected I did not even know it existed. The shamans speak of secrets that we keep, even from ourselves, and I certainly was a master secret keeper.

The eldest Qechua medicine man, Don Manuel Quispe, smiled up at me, and with a giggle and a twinkle acknowledged the difference in our heights. I at once felt seen through his eyes, like the eyes of the magnificent condor peering with such love into me and the design I so creatively constructed. Tears were immediately unleashed. He pressed his medicine bundle, heavy with all the stones used for healing, deep into my heart, transferring all that he had received into his being, from all those that came before. Next, the heavy bundle came to the top of my head, my knees bending to receive it, three times heavily landing.

"Glorify God in your body"
—I Corinthians 20

"Too much mind," he said in Qechua, my Peruvian shaman translating. "Too much thinking, keeping you imprisoned." He pressed the bundle deep into my heart again. "Follow this intelligence."

As the drumming's intensity brought the energies in the room to an ever louder cacophony within me, I was taken deep into a journey to the recesses, nooks, and crannies of my being where I kept myself safe. How did I become my own prisoner? How well I learned to protect myself from myself. The drumming sounded louder within me, expanding me, stretching my hardened walls from deep within a well I had dug.

The shaman now instructed me that at this stage in the journey I was to invoke the animal I would choose to "dismember" me. This sacred animal would take me apart, allowing the most protected of places to become free so that I could see and feel those spaces in between the worlds, in between the perceptions, in between the sensations. In the space lives the knowing; in the space lives the freedom. The indigenous medicine peoples' journey between worlds, the veils so thin they swim through time and space with the fluidity of that eternal river.

I could feel that river bubbling with the intensity of the drums, calling me to realign with the energies of the earth and the heavens, to emerge from my cocoon into all of life, remembering that which I left behind. One of my "power animals," the jaguar, circled me, and another, the condor, flew around me. Each of these magnificent beings have informed me many times before. Would these be my *un*doing? Could I surrender to the power, the forces of nature to *dis*arm me, and would they tear me apart?

As I deepened into my vision quest, I began to feel a soft fabric embracing me, like silk scarves waving around my limbs, over my chest and back, around my head, and across my face like a sweet caress. Ah, the many colored beautiful silk scarves, weaving and flowing between the crevices, under my armpits, around my legs, gently loosening the tight woven patterns of my protective decisions. My architecture was freed from the patterns and shadows of my self-created design. As the scarves wound under my armpits and through the layers of flesh and musculature, my arms gave way and slowly released from my torso, like petals of the most delicate rose, surrendering to that moment when I could no longer hold on. Surrender to the future is oh-so-right in this life cycle and in this design of creation. I was dismembering, releasing from the bonds I created for protection, as every part of me delicately separated from my hardened perceptions. The scarves meandered between my ribs and organs, my pelvis released from my upper torso, and my legs freed from the constraints of having to hold me up.

When no longer bound, I was in space. No longer contained and restricted within my crystallized structure, I emerged into the spaces free. All I could *sense* (although that word no longer seemed an honest one, for I was no longer of the senses) was ever-present space and the me that was no longer kept merging with the All. The energy was like electricity, moving without conduits, without roadways. It kept embracing my awareness and surrounding me in love.

This dismemberment was taking my body's story apart, freeing me from all I created—from this cleverly self-designed structure that secured me so I could move through this lifetime protected within my walls.

My perceptions, my beliefs, my fears, all created a protective covering—a fabric with threads woven so tight, woven deeply through all the layers, so cleverly defined, but certain never to be seen. Yet, I so yearned to be seen.

This place of no boundaries, where information as energy is released begins to *in*form, *re*form and *re*define even my structure.

Tasting the future, being informed by the future as we unravel the hold of the past allows us to widen into new possibility, into creativity, tapping into a river that moves at a pace unencumbered by our old perception. Healing within this new paradigm begins to look and feel very new as we enter through what the shamans call a portal, an opening from which to have new vision and awareness. As we enter into this existence through the cultural histories, the historical histories of all the lineage that preceded us, as well as the eons of physical manifestations that came before, we realize that we are so much more. We remember. The word *remember* can be understood as *re-member*, putting back together that which has been separate, parts living in isolation. Remembering the truth of who we are, as we are, informed by light, ever in formation, ever in creation.

What is your own shamanic story? How have you entered the portals and become unveiled? Taking the body's story apart is incredibly revealing. Perceptions, stories, and beliefs about pain become loosened as we take ourselves back to before we were formed and hardened into crystallized structure, before we partnered with stories that took us far away from the truth of who we are.

As you peer into the places within your body, where is there pain and discomfort? Sometimes we use terms like *stress* or *resistance* but what we are really feeling is fear. How are you wearing your structure? What do those tight places that constrict you and imprison you really tell you? Where in the crevices are the secrets held, in the deepest fabric of the musculature? How have muscles become distorted on and around bones to keep you further hidden in the recesses of your being? Once the energy is freed and your structure begins to move in new ways, unleashing the stories, we put our body back together in a new way.

Remember, evolution is always happening; we are not moving to what was, but on to what is and will be. This body is our vehicle to manifest what we came here to become. Without the fullness of this design, how can we bring in the future and transform into the next best version of humankind? We are not putting ourselves back together in ways that are known. We are evolving and creating, like curious children, as we move through layers with freedom.

The new story that is ready to be rewritten must start at the cellular level. Transformation takes place with the release of old patterns. The neurology is the very last to be informed, for the cells inform the neurology. Remember when you rode a bike for the first time, you did not master that art immediately. Practicing getting on that bike, falling down and getting up, weaving through the streets unsteady, eventually created new pathways of knowledge. Finally, the brain partnered with the cell structure and the musculature and the bones aligned to a new rhythm. Indeed the brain is the last to know, to be informed.

"When we build on belief, we build cement walls around our mobile mental faculties."

—Richard Rose

Now we are ready to embark on our quest for a pain-free, more embodied being, discovering the tools for transformation. Like curious travelers, perhaps archeologists, excited to discover what lies beneath the layers and between the layers, let's find out how we will excavate what lies deep within.

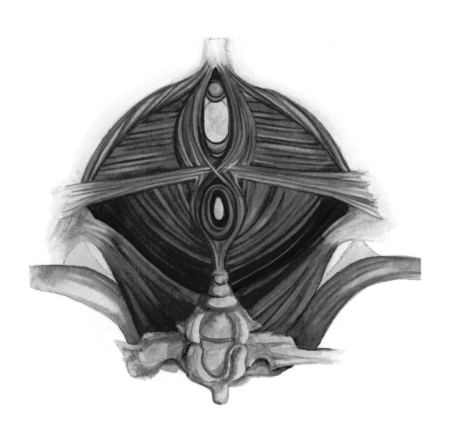

PART TWO

WRITING YOUR BODY'S NEW STORY: PHYSICAL & SPIRITUAL AWAKENING THROUGH STRUCTURAL REALIGNMENT INTEGRATION®

As you work through the exercises in this section,
you will find further resources to support your practice at:
www.corebodywisdom.com
Free videos
Guided Audio Exercises
Workshops, Retreats, and Training

CHAPTER 7

EMBARKING ON THE JOURNEY OF DISCOVERY: THE BASICS OF STRUCTURAL REALIGNMENT INTEGRATION®

*"Inner alignment is the voluntary relation of a human being
with a greater movement. Inner alignment is when I make
myself available; I deepen my listening and my awareness
of the movement I am swimming in."*

—Thomas Hübl

NOW WE ARE ready to discover how following the tangled threads to their source, created through injury and self-protection, can lead to freedom. My method is called Structural ReAlignment Integration® but I will refer to it henceforward as SRI for ease. I developed this protocol after years of working with my own structure and those of hundreds of others. While it is an anatomically based approach, it is energetically sourced. As individual human beings, we are each an energy system and when the flow is blocked we create dysfunction and illness in our bodies.

Through a basic understanding of the anatomy of the perineal area, this protocol offers awareness tools to become intimate with your own imbalance which has led to the creation of distortion and pain. I use imagery and visualization to guide you into the areas of distortion and to help you create space. The series of specific poses, stretches, and movements—each sourced deep within the perineal area—are designed to unravel distorted musculature and rewire your nervous system, allowing you to live a vital, pain free, vibrant life.

Today we have all the information available we need to be the most informed participants in our own care. However, it takes courage and commitment to take our well-being into our own hands. It takes courage and commitment to transform an energy system that is in great stress to one that is capable of "remembering" wholeness and tapping into original energetic movement.

Most people, if asked, would no doubt welcome a chance to be in charge and have partnership in the creation of their well-being. Then again, I have had clients come to me and confide, "This is just too hard. I do not have the time, I do not have the willingness to feel what is buried deep inside. I just want the pain to go away and if surgery will do that so be it." Don't get me wrong, when one needs a hip replacement because there is no other choice, or when the attachments around the knee are so challenged that a knee replacement is mandatory, I am all for it. However, we must still ask, how did the misalignment in the structure create the need for these surgeries? How did the way the body wore its layers of muscles over and on and around the bones create the confusion and the entanglements to begin with? Without an understanding of how we created our imbalances, whether they are structural or emotional, surgery can fix our bodies temporarily but might never support our further awakening nor address how the original imbalance might have created the spiral to surgery, or the need for pharmaceuticals to manage the pain.

> "We are like people locked out of our house, trying to get in by storming the front door. Let us instead quietly slip in by the back door to open the front door from within."
> —Dona Holleman, Yoga Practitioner

Structural ReAlignment Integration provides a map and tools to awaken, transform, and increase proprioception, as well as to enliven the nervous system and cultivate awareness of aspects of our physiology of which we previously had no awareness. When the pelvis—the area of the body on which SRI is centered—finds its correct alignment, muscles release their tension from the bones, muscle tone is normalized, and perception changes. Releasing the distortion in our musculature changes the messages that are firing between the muscle-fiber cells. The correction needs to be made in the fascia, but if the fascial pathways are blocked with muscles that are literally wound up, there can be no undoing of the story created in the muscle fibers.

There are so many ways to hide out, so many distractions and fears that have kept us from ourselves. Again, the commitment and courage to practice, to slow down, and to listen is vital. The experience of SRI, as it begins to unfold, is not just physical. When we become aware of where the blocks are and where the energy is not flowing we can begin to receive information. Energy is light and light is energy in movement. With light, much information from Source is revealed. Remember, light contains information. Light informs. Where we have hidden, shadowy places in the pelvic floor, we have prevented the flow of energy from informing us. This journey involves physical, anatomical, and deep emotional release.

My intention for you is to begin to see the story your body has learned more clearly. Feeling the imbalances creates the space for the possibility of change. Yes, pain does that as well, if we are courageous enough to question our patterns and redefine what we know. This protocol, this journey, is all about making space. That space allows for more possibility, more creativity, more life energy surging.

I am inviting you to return to the source of your beginning in the pelvic floor, to swim through shadows and misaligned fibers, to view and feel the misunderstandings you so fervently believed and protected. This body holds the entire journal of your memories, written in every fiber of your being. Those memories that are real and those that we believed real will appear as you decongest the musculo-cellular fabric. The goal is freedom from pain, certainly. As space is revealed and expands we also open to who we are as energetic beings, we open to destiny, we open to enlightenment.

PRACTICE GUIDELINES

For the exercises in this chapter, all you will need is a yoga mat, a blanket or towel, and a firm chair. If you have a mirror available, do your practice in front of it, as it will be helpful to observe yourself. Wear comfortable clothing and bare feet.

Before you begin, take a moment to read all the way through the instructions so that you know where you will be going. Then return to the beginning and refer to the instructions as often as needed until you are familiar with the sequence. It will seem like a lot of information at first, and you will need to go slowly, but as you learn the basics you will find that they repeat themselves again and again.

I suggest you devote fifteen to thirty minutes each day to your practice. Start with the exercises in this chapter and progress forward to those in the chapters that follow. While it is important to practice the basic stretches daily (the ones I will be sharing in this chapter) you may discover that you can vary your choice of the deeper stretches (see Chapter 9) from day to day. You will notice that although the external posture is different, the inner unraveling at the perineal site is exactly the same.

How long you hold a posture depends on the stretch that you are exploring. Sometimes, three or four breaths with focused intention and presence provides a huge amount of information. Other times you will find that your immersion in the stretch becomes so informative that you are not even paying attention to how long you have been there.

Don't limit your practice to times when you are sitting on your yoga mat. The simple act of standing in line at a bus stop, or sitting in a chair with awareness during a business meeting, when you are on the phone, in the car, or at the movies, can also become your moment-by-moment practice. You take your body everywhere with you and are continually informed as you move. Its tweaks and torques become a measure of when you are out of alignment.

Let's begin by going back to basics—the postures we spend much of each day in but take for granted. We'll begin with standing, then progress to sitting, and lying down. You'll be amazed by how much goes on in these simple, everyday poses and even though it appears no movement is involved, there is movement happening all the time.

STANDING: REDISCOVERING YOUR INNATE ALIGNMENT

We'll start with the most basic demand we place on our body: Standing. The first step in SRI is to relearn how to stand in correct alignment. Our intention is to bring our structure, like a well-supported building, into alignment, supported by gravity not fighting it. Be prepared—when your body is correctly aligned it may feel quite odd! Anyone looking at you, however, will see a person who looks upright and regal.

To begin, let's bring your awareness to some of the ways in which your body may be misaligned.

Stand with your feet hip width apart, which means your feet are below the midline of the hip bones, not the outer edges of your body.

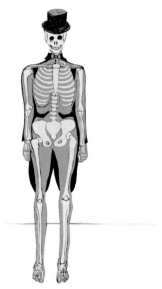

"I'm Feeling So Regal!"

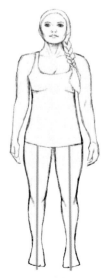

Hip Width Apart

If you look down at your feet, and then trace a line from the space between the second and third toe, up through the center of the knee cap, and on up to your hip bones, you will come to the midline.

Align your feet so that the outer edges (from the base of the baby toe to the heel) are parallel to the outer edges of your yoga mat (or if you are standing on a wood floor, you can line them up with the lines of the panels). Immediately, you will probably feel pigeon-toed and perhaps your knees will feel knock-kneed, as if they are falling in medially. However, you are actually standing straight. Your Achilles tendon is in line with the back of your knee where the hamstring crisscrosses, and then your hamstring extends all the way to the base of the buttocks.

This spot, at the base of the buttocks, is a very significant anatomical location. You may remember Angela Farmer's term "the eye behind the thigh," or the image of the old-fashioned mannequin with the poles holding her up. Bring your awareness to these points on your own body. Again, the "eyes" are not the "sit bones." They are behind the sit bones, lower down from the top of the thighs, at the "smile line" of the buttocks.

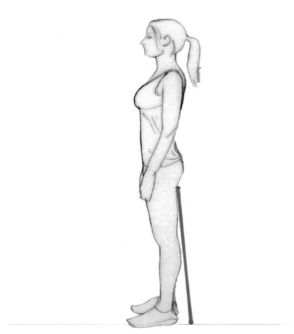

Standing on 4 Legs

If you were to stand with the "eyes" tucked under the pelvis, sucked in, and all the muscle fibers reaching back up and in towards the perineum, the femur bones (the long thigh bones) would be pushed in to the quadriceps muscles and the weight of the body thrust forward off the heels and onto the ball of the toes. Feel that possibility as you tuck the tailbone under and notice how your spine collapses.

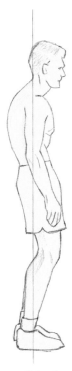

Collapse of the Structure

As you are standing, keep your knees unlocked. By this I mean try to imagine that the tiny patella bone has a little space behind it.

What I suggest is that with slightly bent knees you bring your fingertips around the patella bone and gently pull it forward away from the capsule behind it. Holding on to the bone, if you push the leg bones strongly back, you will feel what a lot of people experience as hyperextension of the knees. Keeping the muscles all around the knees soft is difficult for a lot of people. As the femur, shin, and pelvic bones are pushed forward when the tail tucks under, the knees feel responsible for pulling these bones back in order to keep the body upright. All the anatomy can do is demand that the little patella bones (knee caps) and the femurs and the shin bones suck into the back of the leg. The result is hyperextended knees.

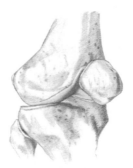

Freedom Behind the Kneecaps

Another result of pushing the pelvis forward and hyperextending the knees is that the arches collapse. With your knees locked, look down at your feet. If you are not standing on the outside line of the feet (from the base of the baby toe all the way to the outside of the heel) the feet are asked to hold the building up without a chance to be in anatomical integrity. All these tiny bones are being pulled and tugged by the muscles of the legs and we lose the ability to stand on the entire base of the foot.

As you practice this, don't forget to breathe. And don't work too hard— you are actually *un*working, unraveling the congested musculature.

What does an aligned body look like? Imagine a circle around the crown of your head, and then a circle around the perineal body. These two circles should be perfectly aligned. With your pelvis thrust forward, notice that your head is thrust forward, with the chin dropped, and these circles cannot be lined up.

Do you have a rounded area that feels like a lump at the base of the neck? Those are the vertebrae that are being pulled back as the weight of the skull droops forward and down. As a result, with the pelvis thrust forward, the vertebrae and the discs are skewed and torqued.

Once again, notice if there is one side of your body that you tend to fall into. This exacerbates the dilemma of achieving balance and having two legs to stand on. As you create space in the floor of the pelvis you will begin to have the space to lift the upper torso out of this droopy side and extend that side's leg out of the pelvis. Then your other leg will get the message that it has a job to do as well. Muscles pulling across the pelvis take the weight off that other leg (the pelvic and femur bones being pulled into the droopy side).

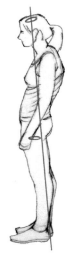

Pathways Obstructed

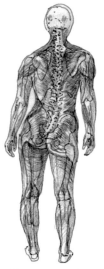

"Droopy Right"

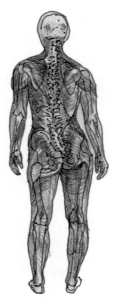

"Droopy Left"

Keeping your knees soft, not locked, slightly bent, let's focus on the alignment of your perineal circle, using the clockface metaphor I introduced in
chapter 1. Remember, 12 o'clock is behind the genitals, 6 is in front of the
anus, 3 is on the right side, and 9 on the left.

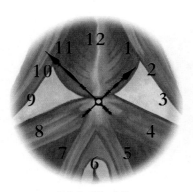

Male Clockface

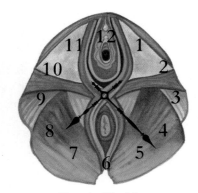

Female Clockface

Let's experiment with what happens to that circle as you change your posture. If you push the leg bones forward and have your weight slide into the

front of your legs, the fibers at 6, 5, and 4 (the bottom back right quadrant of the clock) and 6, 7, 8 (the bottom back left quadrant of the clock) are pulled under. The shape of the perineum is compromised, preventing the energy from reaching into the back of the perineum, and thus into the back of the sacrum and the spine. The light is unable to travel freely, the nervous system is under stress, and our physical body that houses the light energy is compromised. The cells are forced to run interference, the energy is diverted and searching for a free path.

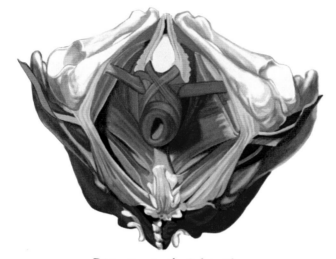

Distortion in the Pelvic Floor

I tend to think of the perineum as a living, breathing, pulsating entity, and in describing it I'll often refer to certain points on the circle "looking" down toward the feet or up toward the nose. What I mean by this is that the circle tilts up and down. As you stand, now, bring your attention to the front of the perineum, behind the genitals (12 o'clock) and allow it to gently release down so that the whole circle is in alignment with the crown circle. If you tuck the pelvis under, what happens to the front of the perineum (12 o'clock)? It is lifted and tilted up towards your chest. If you put your fingertips lightly on the bony part of your pubic bone and draw your fingertips down toward the floor stretching the muscle fiber over the bone, you will bring the front of the perineum back into alignment (you may feel that you have created a deeper arch in your low back).

Now, let's look at how you are standing. Your weight should release into the back body so that you are standing on the heels as well as the balls of the toes (however, you are not leaning back). In order to bring the body back to standing on the heels as well as the balls of the toes, and elongate the exaggerated low back (lumbar) arch, the muscles of the sacrum must release off the back body so that we have space between and behind the sacral bones and between the numerous layers of muscle fiber. This is tricky, for the back of the perineal clock numbers must expand open from the center of the perineal body, fanning out of the middle of the virtual clock like the feathers in a peacock's tail.

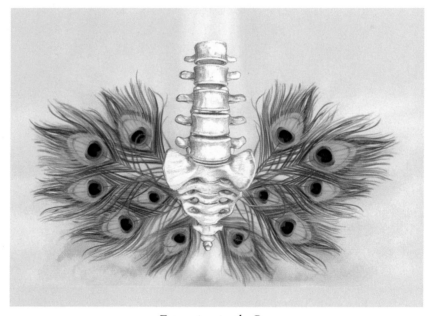

Expansion in the Base

Experience that expansion, and as you do so, you will feel how tangled and raveled the muscle fibers have been, as they retreat under and up into the center of the perineum. Noticing how the pelvis is pushed forward, and which side is drooping lower, will guide you to the place where the muscle fibers are most contracted. If you tend to drop into the right side of your body, then it will be the fibers at 6, 5, and 4 that will be pulled more forcibly under. And if you tend to drop into your left side, it will be the fibers at 6, 7, and 8. Find that place on the clockface deep within your own body: this is where you need to focus to begin the undoing process.

When you open up the back numbers of the perineum, the sacrum is freed from the pelvis, and the pelvis relaxes backward, creating space between the top of the thighs and the bottom of the pelvic bones. This is called the root of the thigh, where the femur bone and the bottom of the pelvis meet. When there is space between the pelvis and the top of the legs, the muscles on the femur bones soften and have room to move on and around the bones. The previously congested spaces around the perineum begin to expand as you focus your breath into those spaces. The fibers begin to unravel and inform more muscle-fiber cells that this is the correct place to live. Eventually, the message gets through to your neurology and the new alignment becomes more familiar.

Now, let's turn our attention to the abdominal muscles, specifically those behind the pubic bone. With the front of the perineum (12) facing downward, what tends to happen is that the back (6) rises up, creating that deeper arch in the low back. To be in alignment, they both need to be at the same level, and it is your abdominals that will help you bring 6 down into alignment with 12 while the fibers on either side of 6 remain open.

When we hear the term *abdominals* (or *abs*) we tend to think of those "six-packs" we see on bodybuilders and models. But the abdominals actually start much lower down. Place your fingertips on the fleshy area right above the hard pubic bone. Gently, with the tiniest amount of pressure, push your fingers inward toward your back body. You will feel a slight pressure move into the sacrum. In the SRI exercises, I'll be asking you each time to move your abdominals into the back body, and this is what I mean. I sometimes call it the "belly in the back."

Important note: If you push too hard, you will force those number lines between 6, 5, 4 and 6, 7, 8 under and up into the perineum, creating a tucked under feeling, as if sucking your buttocks under your spine.

Immediately the sacral muscles elongate off the sacral bone as 6, 5, 4, and 6, 7, and 8 expand all of the muscles at the base of the buttocks. With both 12 and 6 looking down, your circle is now in alignment with the earth.

Your sit bones are way back behind you and the "eyes behind the thighs" are far back, as if those mannequin poles would drop straight down behind your heels.

You probably feel like your butt is way back in the breeze as some of my clients say, and you may even feel as if you are coming off the ball of the toes because you are so firmly rooted in your heels. Crawl your toes out of the back of the arch of your feet, which lengthens your arch, and brings the weight onto the ball of the toes as well as the heels.

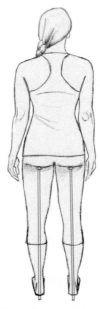

Standing on 4 Legs

Your perineum is now free to open wider, expanding your whole pelvic floor and providing a more spacious base for your structure. Your quadriceps muscles will begin to soften and the femur bones behind them release toward the back of the leg where they belong.

Anatomically, the movement of your buttocks this far back is the correct alignment and it yet feels so foreign. Also, you will feel quite confused as your bones are becoming free from the tight hold of the musculature. Your balance will feel strange. Like most of people I work with, you may be thinking, "This cannot be right!" But remember, what you believed to be "right" until now is the result of being informed by years of misalignment. Proprioceptors in the muscle-fiber cells have informed your neurology and your structure has learned a posture that incorporates unfortunate distortion. When we make changes in alignment, our brain and its neurology, says, "Not right." But the brain only knows what it has been taught over and over again. So be patient, for there is more changing here than just your spinal alignment.

When you are standing in correct alignment, the center of the perineal circle, where the hands of the clock meet, will be directly in line with the center of the circle above your crown circle.

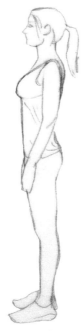

Correct Alignment

When the muscles let go of their stranglehold on the bones, the legs elongate out of the pelvis with ease into the earth and the upper torso becomes free of the collapse that was caused by tucking the pelvis under. Spinal muscles engage and elongate, lifting the upper torso out of the pelvis. The legs now have more space as the congestion in the musculature unravels.

You are now freer to wiggle your upper torso way out of the droopy side and stretch your opposite leg into the earth. I like to think of the legs like giant screws, unscrewing from the pelvis and screwing deeper into the earth.

You will feel lighter on the droopy side leg, which is great as you now have the other leg to stand on. The congestion that is freeing up at the top and around the upper thigh of the droopy leg will allow this leg to emerge out of the pelvis little by little.

For those who practice yoga, here's an image you may find helpful: standing in correct alignment, the lift of the upper torso all the way out of the base, with the upper chest expanding and space created in the low back, is a true backbend.

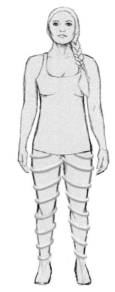

Unscrewing the Leg bones

Now that you have created more space between the legs and the pelvis, your abdominals are free to stretch up and out. Place your fingertips into the space at the root of the thighs, between the front of the thigh bone and the bottom of the pelvis. If you press inward, you can lift the abdominals from beneath and raise them up off the legs. Once again, you have more freedom to crawl the legs deeper out of the pelvic floor and into the earth.

Imagine that your hands could go deeper, inside your body, and lift those abdominals up. The psoas muscle on the inner upper thighs comes into action. The engaged muscles up the front and back of the spine are free to elongate the upper torso out of the pelvic floor. The upper chest lifts off the ribcage, creating freedom for the heart and lungs and more space for the diaphragm.

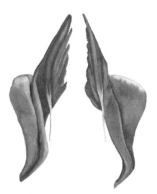

Psoas Musculature

This may feel quite tiring. The erector spinae muscles—the long thick muscles that stretch along the sides of the vertebrae and are attached to the facets of the vertebrae—are not always happy about being stretched.

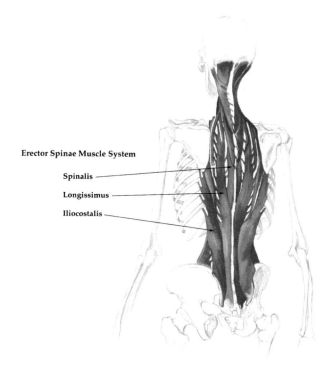

Erector Spinae Muscle System

Spinalis ———

Longissimus ———

Iliocostalis ———

The Erector Spinae

The area in the thoracic spine that becomes rounded as we age starts to elongate as you stretch and spaces are created between the vertebrae. It may feel achy, but this is actually good news because these muscles are lengthening and the bones are responding, literally moving; the discs between the vertebrae are expanding to fill the new spaces. The area in the upper thoracic and the cervical spine that becomes painful and tired when the skull drops so far forward eventually elongates as well, and brings the head back into alignment.

As you practice your standing, you will initially feel more and more confused as more fibers are coming into play to support your realignment. However, each time you realign your pelvis by opening those back numbers, elongating the sacrum so your upper torso can move up and out and your legs can move down and out, you will begin to feel taller.

I suggest practicing this as many times throughout the day as you can. When you are waiting on line anywhere, you have the opportunity to become conscious of your posture. As you wash dishes or brush your teeth, notice how you are standing. And in addition, try to intentionally practice on your mat, two times a day, morning and evening, for five to ten minutes. Move into the stretch and then release, several times, playing with the numbers around your clock. What you may notice, as the muscle fibers stretch, in new ways is tension in places you have not felt before. Please be kind and gentle with yourself because as openings arise, new and deeper patterns reveal themselves. The stretches sometimes change every time you practice, making new space for more movement.

SITTING, SITTING, AND MORE SITTING: DON'T SIT ON THOSE SIT BONES

Standing is perhaps the most difficult place to feel these shifts, so let's move into a seated posture.

Sitting on a firm chair, close to the lip of the seat, first align your feet under the pelvis exactly as you did in the standing posture. The shin bone should be perpendicular to the thigh bone, creating a right angle with your leg bones.

Notice if one foot is more turned out than the other. You will most likely feel pigeon-toed again.

Then bring your awareness to the circle of the perineum. Think of your 12 o'clock as dropping forward on the chair; you will not be leaning toward the back of the seat, collapsing on to the sit bones. If you do lean back gently, what happens to 12? It lifts off the chair and you can feel the collapse (the rounding) of your back body. You will fall toward the back of the seat and the mid-back (the thoracic) will collapse. The head will fall forward and you will find yourself in a seated version of the typical standing posture.

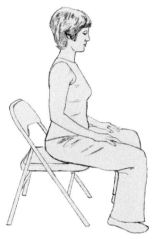

Sitting in Aignment

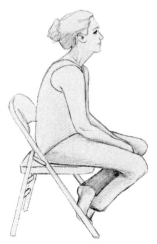

Sitting in Collapse

In this collapsed posture, look at your feet, and notice that your weight is not on the ball of the toes; you are sliding back into the heels, just as in your standing posture. You feel the toes and balls of the toes becoming weightless on the floor. The femurs begin lifting up off the seat toward the ceiling and receding into your pelvis, and only the heels are making slight contact.

Just as in your standing posture, you want the legs to have the freedom to elongate out of the pelvis. When you drop 12 down into the seat, notice how the weight transfers onto your feet. When the femurs are free of the pelvic floor they can stretch out, the lower leg bones elongate and the feet make a connection with the floor. The feet will actually have weight, and can press gently, as if massaging into the floor. Imagine that the floor is made of soft earth or sand, and you can push the feet through the floor. Now, you are weight-bearing in a sitting position, as you are when standing.

Notice also how when you allow 12 to lift up and you fall back onto the tailbone, the fibers around the back edges of the perineum get sucked under, as do the muscle fibers at 6, 5, 4 and 7, 8, 9, under the upper thighs. Sitting more on the sit bones here will congest the very base of the spine, leaving the energy imprisoned, preventing the flow. The spine will never be able to climb up and out.

> "Posture should be steady and comfortable."
> —Yoga Sutras of Patangali

As you did in the standing pose, with 12 looking down toward the lip of the seat, place your fingers above the pubic bone, and gently press the abdominals into the back body. The anatomical response is that the sacral muscle fibers elongate 6 o'clock down into the seat and your base (the perineal circle) is planted on the chair.

You can help the opening movement by placing your fingertips under your upper thighs, close to where the thigh meets the buttocks, the base of the sacrum and the coccyx. Reaching as close as possible to the place where the thigh meets your pelvic floor on the right side, with the fingers of your right hand, gently fan out the 6, 5, and 4 fibers. Visualize those stretching fibers beginning in the center of the perineum, stretching the fabric of the musculature all the way towards the far right side of your chair. This side now feels much more expanded. 3 o'clock now feels wider, more open, and farther away from 9 o'clock. Repeat the same with the fingers of your left hand, so that 9 o'clock also opens with the expansion of 6, 7, and 8.

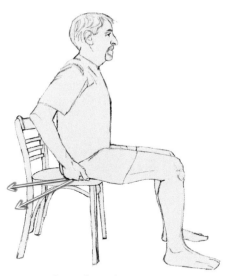

Spreading the Numbers

You may notice that one side is much more congested and has more dif-
ficulty breathing and stretching out of the middle of the perineum. You may
also notice which side is heavier on the chair, and this may mirror the same
droopy side you noticed in your standing posture. Look down at your arches
as well and see the collapse. Using your fingers, expand those fibers out from
the perineum on your dropped side and notice whether you feel more weight
on the opposite side.

When I sit, since my right side is my droopy side, I always elongate those
fibers under my right buttock so that I can grow my upper torso and my
femur out of that collapse. Opening my left fibers with my left fingers, I now
feel my left "eye under the thigh" heavier if not equal on the seat.

Remember to breathe. Feel your breath, like a river, flowing through the
crown all the way down through the perineum to the base of the pelvis and
through the chair into the earth.

This sitting posture becomes like a squat on a chair (an idea we will explore in more depth in chapter 9). When you witness a young child in a squat,
he or she is literally hanging through the open perineum and 12 o'clock is
dropped forward easily. Not so for those of us who have spent years tucking 6
o'clock under, with the fibers all pulling and skewing around the anus, lifting
12 o'clock up toward the nose.

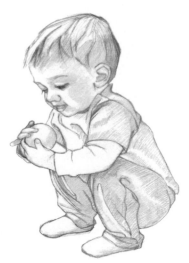

"Eyes" Way Back

The baby has space between the femur and the bottom of the pelvis. For most of us, this is not the case. With the lift of 12 there is no space at the top of the thighs for the upper torso to rise up and out. In cultures where adults continue to squat, the pelvic floor is open and the spine climbs straight up and out.

Still sitting in your chair, look at your inner legs close to the pelvic floor as well as the inner thighs and the inner knees all the way down to your feet. The flesh on the inner thighs tends to roll inward closing off the space between the bottom of the pelvis and the upper thigh bone (the root of the thigh). Looking at your knees you may see them falling inward. And it is always a very different story on each side.

Expanding your back numbers around the perineum might have caused the numbers around the front quadrants (12, 1, 2, and 12, 11, 10) to roll inwards, with the flesh and muscles around the upper thighs and inner legs collapsing inward as well. Opening and creating space in one region will have repercussions in another because all these fibers are connected. Every muscle fiber in our body is connected to every other.

To support the unraveling and opening of the fibers around the front of the clockface, place your thumb on each hand into the crease between the thigh and the bottom of the pelvic bone. Your other fingers will be splayed open around the upper thighs and out to the side of the thigh. Breathing all the way into the perineum, visualize the breath streaming from the dot of the circle where the hands of the clock meet, and opening the fibers between 12 and 1, then between 1 and 2. Now, do the same on the left side—direct your breath, like that river, between 12 and 11, and between 11 and 10. Your fingers will gently follow that opening through all the layers of muscle fiber, so that you can, with your breath, expand, from the center of the perineum, the outer layers of flesh that your hands are touching.

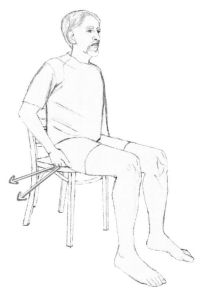

Expanding the Base

Look around the clockface, internally, and at each number, notice if you feel connection with the chair underneath you. Remember, this is a journey to unravel the areas that you may not have any connection with at all. Noticing areas of numbness around the perineum, that don't allow you to feel connected to the chair, is vital. Pain in a hip, in the sacrum, or elsewhere, can be retraced to areas all around the perineum—often, those areas are where the congestion has created "dead zones." What we cannot feel and see becomes very enlightening.

Once again, go to the underside of the thighs with your fingers and expand those lower back numbers all the way to the outside of the seat. Does this now feel different?

With more of your numbers on the chair, 12, 1, 2, and 3, and 12, 11, 10, and 9, as well as 6, 5, and 4, and 6, 7, and 8 you can begin to feel the spine elongating up and out of the pelvis, as are the leg bones extending out so that the feet deepen into the floor even more. Just as I described standing as a true backbend, both sitting and standing are an eternal inner squat!

The same would be true for sitting in your car. If you are sitting forward onto the front of the perineum, with the "belly in the back," and with all your numbers in contact with the seat, you will probably have to change the position of the rearview mirror. You are taller. You will have to tilt it so that your eyes can now see what is happening behind your car. If you lean back, as if sitting on a couch curled into your back body, the mirror will need to be adjusted downwards so your eyes can align with it.

I pull the back of my seat far forward so that my 12 o'clock can drop down easily and with my low and mid back supported in this forward position I remind my abdominals behind the pubic bone to gently move into my back body as 12 o'clock peers down into the seat between my legs. I am always doing both of these movements together. The perineal body sinking through the soft fabric of the seat, I widen my numbers with my fingers (at a traffic light). The muscles on the thighs begin to relax, the center of the perineum melts. My spine climbs higher and with my hands on the steering wheel I can feel the extension as I wiggle up and out, getting taller and taller. Hence the need to tilt the rearview mirror again and again.

Whenever you are sitting—whether in a movie theater, at your desk, or on a plane with those horrible seats and head rests, it is all the same. You may need to roll up your jacket, or your sweater behind your low back to support your lumbar spine. You always want to be sitting forward on 12 o'clock, and expand all of the fibers out in every direction around that perineal circle. You want to feel your leg bones getting heavier and heavier, dropping into the seat beneath you.

Remember, do not sit on those sit bones!

LYING DOWN

Lying on the floor is an excellent opportunity to feel your alignment. The floor does not lie! (You may want to have a rolled up washcloth for under your neck if your chin tends to lift up and shorten your cervical area).

Lie down on a firm surface, such as a yoga mat or a thin carpet. Bend your knees, placing your feet hip-width apart. The center of your feet should be in alignment with the mid line of your pelvic bones not the outer edges of your body. You may notice how you are more connected to the floor on one side of your body; your sacrum may melt deeper into the ground on one side than the other. The opposite side may not feel connected to the floor at all. Notice if one foot is turned out more than the other and once again realign your feet as you did while standing and sitting. Your Achilles tendon in this lying down position will be directly in line with the eye behind your thigh. You may feel slightly pigeon-toed as before.

The base of your spine, where the tailbone emerges, should be on the floor, as should the entire sacral bone. When the front of the perineum (at 12 o'clock) is looking down toward your feet, not pushed down but gently breathed downwards between the legs, the base of your spine touches the floor. Yes, you may feel more of a lumbar curve at this juncture. Be patient, for you will elongate the spine momentarily and create the space in the lumbar necessary to extend out of your base, just as you did standing and sitting. You will notice, as we continue working with SRI, that it always comes back to the same movements.

With closed eyes, bring your meditative awareness into the floor of the pelvis. Breathe deeply, down into the base. Send your inner vision into your perineal area and while the base of the buttocks and the connection at the inner upper thigh may be elevated off the floor, we want the fibers at 6, 5, and 4, and 6, 7, and 8 to expand outward away from the center point of the perineal circle. You can use your fingers to open these fibers under the thighs, close to the pelvic floor.

With those strands opening, the base of the spine and the base of the buttocks are free to release downward, melting into the floor. As in our standing and sitting posture, if 12 o'clock is lifted up, the strands around the back of the perineal body are tucked under.

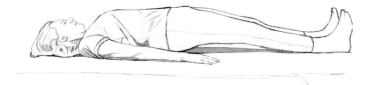

Pelvis in Stress

This will cause the leg bones to be lifted away from the floor and jammed up into the quadriceps, and the base of the spine and the base of the buttocks are not in contact with the floor.

Which side of your sacrum do you feel is dropped closer to the ground? Does it feel like the same side as in your standing and sitting posture? With your fingers underneath the base of the buttocks, close to the area between the coccyx and the back of the upper thigh, open these numbers and feel the stretch of the fibers elongating out of the perineum. Once again, one side is likely to be more resistant. Becoming aware of the imbalance is the doorway to making change and freedom.

Breathe your ribcage downwards away from your chest. You can put your hands gently on the lower ribs and feel the ribs moving downwards with your exhalations. Your scapulae (shoulder blades) will drop off your back body into the floor as your attention, your internal gaze, looks to the perineum.

Notice, once again, whether your legs, the base of the buttocks, and the base of the sacrum are elevated. If they are, your 12 o'clock is lifted up. Put your fingertips gently on the flesh of the pubic bone and softly guide these fibers away from your upper body through your legs. You will feel space created right above the pubic bone. When you drop 12 o'clock away from your nose and toward your feet, the ribcage tends to pop up, creating that deeper lordosis (curve) in your lumbar spine.

Once again, put your hands on your lower ribs as you breathe and guide the breath into your pelvic floor. Allow the ribs under your hands to relax away from your upper chest toward your legs. Imagine your exhalations as a river of warm light filling your back body and the ribs sliding towards your pelvis. You will be able to fill the area at the base of your shoulder blades with the breath and the lumbar region directly below as well. Allow the breath to soften the muscles in the lumbar area so that they fall toward the floor. The intention here is to have more of your front body surrendering into the back body, like the surrender into the hammock, so that you are making more contact with the floor.

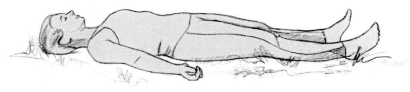

Releasing Into the Earth

There will always be a temptation to squeeze your pelvic floor sphincters, an unconscious movement that we learned very early on in order to protect the floor of the pelvis. If you notice that you are contracting the sphincters, then breathe into these spaces. Be aware of the tenderness and the stories that may be held in this area. This is the place we were birthed into with all the karma and cultural history that came along.

It is a good practice to notice how often you squeeze the anal and genital sphincters as you go about your day. Also, if you can become more cognizant of your tendency to collapse into one side more than another, you will begin to connect not only physical stories that have crystallized your structure but emotional ones that have protected you as well. I have discovered that the fear I experienced growing up in my home, had me contract deeply into the right side of the perineum. Protecting myself, my body wore the result of my terror.

As you lie on the floor, notice, without judgment, if one side is more challenging to release. Breathe. Receive the information. If there is discomfort, can you allow this to be present as you are being informed? As you fall gently into the earth with the front of the perineum, your leg bones heavier, as you breathe your exhalations down into the base, as you allow your shoulder blades to melt off your structure into the floor beneath you, place your arms with bent elbows alongside your upper torso with your lower arms and fingers pointed up to the ceiling. Put some weight into your elbows and immediately feel the ribcage want to raise up. Breathe the ribs gently down and pressing your upper arms into the floor, walk your shoulders one at a time away from your pelvic floor, elongating your upper back out of your base as you keep breathing 12 o'clock downwards allowing your sacral bones to gently release underneath you into the earth. You now have taken some of the excess lumbar curve out of your back and become taller once again as the spine emerges out of the pelvis.

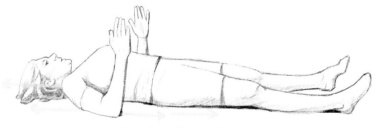

Crawling Out of the Base

Your breath is your connection to the divine river, the rise and fall of the waves of light informing and releasing old patterns. These moments you are committed to feeling are precious ones. Honor your past, for it has certainly served you well in protecting you from your pain both physically and emotionally. As you unravel your distortions, feeling more space where tension and emotion have been hiding out, your future expands before you. Like a snake shedding its skin to emerge anew, we emerge out of the congestion to meet ourselves in our truest alignment, open to possibility.

For further resources to support your inquiry, including videos, guided audio exercise, and more visit:

www.corebodywisdom.com

CHAPTER 8

VISUALIZATIONS
AND MEDITATIONS

"Meditation must begin with the body."
—B.K.S. Iyengar

AS HUMANS, WE are blessed with both outer and inner vision. We can perceive the physical world around us, but we also have a rich inner world of imagination that we can harness in service of our own healing and growth. Throughout these pages, I have repeatedly invited you to engage your inner vision and "look" inside your body, journeying deep into the pelvic floor. Wise teachers for millennia have understood the power of symbols and metaphors, and today the technique of focusing on specific images has become a respected and well-researched healing modality known as guided imagery. One of the foremost researchers in this field, Belleruth Naparstek, explains that the practice "has the built-in capacity to deliver multiple layers of complex, encoded messages by way of simple symbols and metaphors."[61]

Structural ReAlignment Integration incorporates imagery and the power of inner vision into all of its movements. You've already encountered this when I've asked you to envision the perineal clockface or the peacock tail fanning out from the center of the perineum. These images do indeed send messages to your cells, imprinting them with new information. To help you develop your powers of inner perception, in this chapter I will offer a series of visualizations that you can do in a meditative state. These are images that have been evocative for me and my clients; however, you may discover or create your own images that prove to be effective in opening the doors of your perception.

The power of imagery to inform us is oftentimes magical. We become like an artist in our mind, painting pictures that allow us to step off the edges of linear time and into spaces otherwise unknown to us. Visually, we can take journeys through the layers of time, space, structure, and rhythm. Recently, I had a powerful experience of this in the fitting environment of an art gallery. I was at an exhibition called *Painting the Modern Garden: From Monet to Matisse,* which included all of the painters from the Impressionist School who, through their love of gardening, began painting the floral majesty of the divine presence. I had no idea that for some of these painters they were gardeners first. As I witnessed the divinity before me, I was taken through veils of time into these gardens, feeling the artist as he captured the divine essence of the flower with his brush.

My journey through the galleries, with the heart, passion, and soul of these artists informing me, allowed me to drop back in time. These messengers of divine beauty, in their expanded consciousness, awakened me with their sight. The profound love of God's beauty that was exquisitely received through every cell in their being was now vibrating through my cellular memory. I stood before Monet as he stood before his garden, feeling the deep honor and the gratitude for him being the conduit of this magnificent transmission. My eyes filled with tears as I felt, deep within my essential truth, the beauty that the artist had brought into this world, through time, without time.

> "Dis-covering is un-covering that which is already there."
> —**Dona Holleman**

The hours I spent walking down those painted forested paths bursting with life allowed me to feel them coming to life within me—no longer layers of paint. This is the kind of experience I hope you will have as we take a journey through the layers of your divine structure all the way to the source of your beginning. This body is informed through all of the layers of patterning, of beliefs, of traumas, of love often not remembered. We will embark together on the journey back into the base, where we first landed at the site that became the perineum.

Before we begin, a few words about how I use the term "meditation." For some, the very word may conjure up a whole host of expectations that might put you off. Meditation is an ancient spiritual modality, written about in Indian scriptures more than five thousand years ago. You do not need to go into an ashram and sit in silence for days at a time to meditate. In a broader sense, meditation is simply a time to quiet the senses and create a space to receive deep silence. Some form of this is found in most spiritual disciplines, and in religious services, there is always a time to sit in reflection. It is in the quiet, in the spaces in between the noise and the constant input from our own mind and all that surrounds us, that we become aware of information behind the senses. In these silences, we can have moments of creative awareness and sparks of intelligence not previously experienced.

Meditation doesn't just mean sitting still. Taking a walk in the woods or around your neighborhood can be a meditation as you become immersed in the world around you. Or you might like sitting in a park in quiet reflection and contemplation. Swimming in a pool or in the sea, for some, is a meditative experience, as is reading lines in a book that have you in awe so that you have to keep rereading them for they are so profound to you.

Eventually, you will be able to practice the visualizations I will be sharing with you in any of these meditative states. To begin, though, I'd suggest you sit still or lie down, in a quiet and comfortable place where you will be undisturbed. Read through the entire visualization before attempting to practice and then you can break it down into smaller parts and refer back to the description as often as needed.

Although you are practicing in stillness, I will be asking you to bring attention to various parts of your body, and sometimes to relax or release tension in certain areas. I will also be bringing your attention to your breath. Breathing is an important aspect of meditation. Right now, wherever you are reading these words, take deep, slow breaths to create inner space.

"Keep on walking. Don't buy what the mind wants to sell you."

—Thomas Hübl

I want to guide you through some patterns of imagery that you can visualize to become more intimate with your pelvic floor. For light to *in*form us, to *re*form us, we need to enter the visual, kinesthetic river of light and love. Anatomy on the page can be exquisite but two-dimensional; anatomy brought alive through inner awareness will inform us and educate us as to our history in a different way. Yes, there are illustrations to refer to, which may help you picture what I'm describing and understand the anatomy. However, keep returning to your inner canvas, like the artist, and paint your own pictures that will resonate for you. I love to play with image and metaphor, and in the pages that follow you will see the canvas of my imagination laid out. No doubt some of the images will be more powerful and evocative for you than others—choose the ones that you like, or create your own. I hope that among these suggested visuals and stories you will find at least a few that will support your meditative journey to seeing and feeling places within the pelvic floor that perhaps have been lying in the shadows.

My wish for you is that through this discovery you experience your deepest connection to a higher resonance field—tapping into vibrations that inform more of who you are. Let's begin.

SURRENDERING INTO THE SACRED HAMMOCK

Lying down on the floor or on your bed, close your eyes. Imagine you are stepping outside your body and standing beside yourself. Picture yourself lying in a hammock. This attitude of "stepping outside" and observing oneself is sometimes called the perspective of the witness. In this practice, you are witnessing your body in the hammock at the same time as you feel your body in the hammock. While you see yourself hanging, feel yourself dropping deeper and deeper with every breath into the fabric of this divine net. The fabric is tightly woven to hold the very essence of your being, allowing you to melt your divine structure into the hammock of safety where you are completely held, surrendering and releasing all tension.

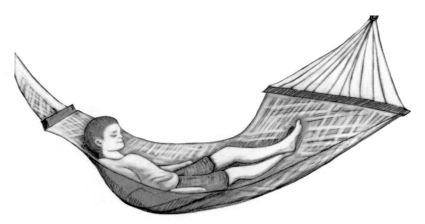

Surrender into the Back Body

As you look at "you" from the perspective of the witness, seeing yourself dropping slowly into the hammock, feel, at the same moment, the letting go of the tension in your buttocks, your back, your legs, your arms, neck, and skull. Breathe delicately and completely into your back body, for you are surrendering into the care and support you have always wanted.

As you watch yourself falling sweetly into the fabric of the hammock, experience that letting go and observe the huge C-curve that your body makes, the heaviness of the buttocks, the back, and the legs sinking you deeper, with no need to hold yourself up.

As you breathe deeper, your exhalations guiding you in the river of life's light, tension releases, and any need to know if this fabric will indeed support you melts away. Notice where you are holding tension, where your past habits of constricting and contracting muscles are keeping you from those places you protected and did not want to feel.

Where are you squeezing and tightening, protecting yourself from letting go? Pause here and let the breath seep deeply into one of these spaces that is tightly held, allowing it to receive breath and then to expand. The fabric of the hammock caresses you ever more as you surrender even deeper.

"A silent body is a body that has a natural dignity."
—Dona Holleman

Allow your pelvis to drop deeper with every exhale. Feel the breath filling your sacrum, like gentle fingers of light. Visualize the light widening the two halves of the sacrum. Imagine there is a space to fall right through and in-between the two halves of the sacrum.

Release the sphincters in the pelvic floor, noticing, as you carefully release, where around the pelvis there is tension, protection like a cloak, a veil that keeps you hiding from yourself. We have each built our fortress of safety deep inside and as a result have abandoned ourselves, leaving behind our essential nature.

As you breathe into your back body, the fabric of your musculature, the many layers of muscle, drops off behind you. Your back body is your hammock. It is always there and as you breathe, you are held. The tension releases, surrendering you ever more deeply.

Visualize the front of the perineum dropping deeply into the fabric of the hammock and feel your upper thighs at the base of the buttocks let go. Your quadriceps and all the other muscles on your legs fall away and the bones are held by the fabric of the musculature in your back body, the hammock you are always lying in.

Let yourself melt even deeper.

If you wanted to lift yourself out of the hammock, it would not be an easy feat. Lifting your sacrum out of the depth of the release would require a tightening and a tension in buttocks and the pelvic floor.

As you continue to let go, and your firm, tight buttock muscles unwind, feel the base of the buttocks and the upper thighs descend.

With your breath, allow the sacrum to fall back into your net. Now, I invite you to journey with your meditative awareness inside your body and down to the pelvic floor. Look deep inside at the perineal area, between the anus and the genitals. Picture the muscle fibers that have been retreating up into the perineum, distorting this exquisite flower, like petals wrinkled, sucked up, hidden from view. With your breath expanding into the perineum, now see the petals of that flower blooming right out of the center of the perineum.

Focus on the centermost point of the perineal body. As you feel this sacred space and visualize the clockface superimposed on its circle, can you imagine light emanating from the midpoint out like a fan to every point around the circle?

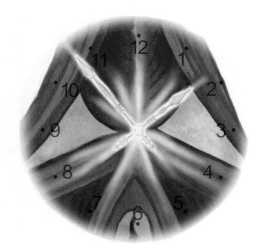

The "En Lightened" Perineum

There are places that are constricted more than others. Trace with your inner vision, as if you have a flash light and can see, as well as feel, where the shadows and numb areas reside.

Remember, the base in the floor of your pelvis is the home of safety. But as a child, in protection mode, you contracted and pulled away from your original wounds. As you witness your letting go into the imaginary fabric of your back body, your hammock, it may bring up old feelings, as well as feelings of numbness, for those are feelings too. When we do not have a feeling in an area and say we are numb that often indicates that there has been a decision to cut off, for protection. Under the numbness is a warehouse of feeling.

Breathe and explore.

As you breathe your sacred light from the centermost point in the circle out to every number, feel the lines of light expanding and melting, widening your pelvis. Fall deeper into your hammock.

Do you feel that you have enough space in your own base? Or does it feel, as you breathe and let go, that this sacred vessel is too tight? Do you sense that there is anger, shame, fear, frustration, or sadness as you explore and fall into your back body? Do you feel that you can drop even more? Or are you pulling up and retreating from this power source?

As emotions arise, breathe into the spaces that are revealing these feelings. Let the body inform you. Don't try to figure out anything as you breathe and notice and feel. The journey into the base, into the perineum, holds much mystery. Honor your intention as you explore with loving compassion.

> *"The mountain is the mountain,*
> *And the path unchanged since the old days.*
> *Verily what has changed is my own heart."*
> **—Sally Kempton**

WAVING THE BREATH, ROLLING THE BELLY

Let's explore how the breath, like a gentle river, moves through our innermost channel, following the length of the spinal column and calming the nervous system.

As you sit on a chair, with the pelvic floor open, imagine the numbers all around the clockface of the perineum unfurling like petals of a flower opening. Focus on the central point, that dot in the center of the clock and then feel the spaces widening, expanding, to bring your base fuller and more present beneath you. As we did in the sitting exercise (p. 139), you can use your fingers beneath your thighs to spread the skin and flesh and muscle away from the midpoint of the perineal area.

See the front of the perineum (12 o'clock) dropping onto the seat, with 6 dropping as well. Move the abdominals in toward your back body. Elongate your femur bones as if the kneecap is moving over your toes. Feel your feet engage the earth and your spinal muscles elongate your upper torso out of your base.

Visualize looking down into the perineum from above, opening the petals of the flower with your every breath, inhaling all the way down into the base and exhaling the river of breath like a gentle stream through the perineum. Imagine it opening out like a starburst, like a perfect circle of light emanating from the center and all the way below under your body and through the chair. The cushion of the chair now becomes like the hammock, the place in which you are being received. Your legs, the muscles on the under thighs, are being cradled into the chair.

With your streaming breath, let go of the sphincters in the pelvic floor. Feel the weight of your bones deepening through the soft musculature into the chair.

Feel 12 letting go even more, and with your fingertips on the flesh over the pubic bone, feel that muscle slide off the bone. With the abdominals gently looking into the sacrum, feel 6 release through the chair as well.

Now there is space between the top of the thighs and the bottom of your pelvis. There is room for your abdominal muscles to begin to roll up from behind the pubic bone, like a cushioned rolling pin, toward your upper chest.

You may now feel more centered in that channel that carries energy through the perineum from the crown circle at the top of your head and back up. As you breathe, wave the breath all the way out of the base, exhale by exhale up the spine, continuing to sink your leg bones through the chair. Deepen your breath into the base and your buttocks into the chair, as if you were going to sink right through. Allow the ribcage to fall with every exhalation. With closed eyes, the breath fills the entire pelvic bowl; every muscle-fiber cell fills with energy.

Energy is movement. Energy is what moves us. Drop your tongue from the upper palette, and as you breathe, feel the breath move all the way into the interior walls of the neck, back where the muscle fibers hold the tongue deeply into the back of the throat. Feel that space at the base of your skull (the occiput), right behind the ears, the interior of your neck widening, and see and feel the movement of the river all the way up through the two hemi-spheres of the brain and up through the crown.

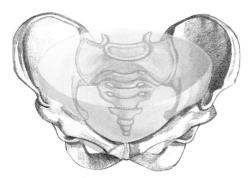

The Pelvis as a Bowl

Back and forth, up and down, the breath waves and breathes you. As you are surrendering through the layers of confusion and congestion, it is unwinding ancient patterns and stories that have kept you hidden even from yourself.

A SEA ANEMONE

Another image that I find to be helpful is that of a sea anemone, with waving fiber-like tentacles undulating calmly in the moving water. Imagine the anemone upside down, with its fibers reaching toward the ocean floor.

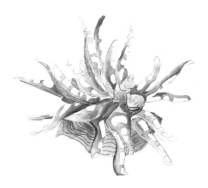

The Perineal Body as a Sea Anemone

Now, closing your eyes, superimpose this image onto the perineal body. Feel the undulating streamers of fiber releasing with the gentle motion of the sea. Imagine your breath becoming the gentle waves of the ocean, traveling between the fibers that are curled and twisted around each other. The flowing breath separates the fibers. Spaces expand so that the water, filled with information, can move into areas of darkness, shadowy unknown places. The river of light, gently seeps through the crevices, bringing with it so much hidden information. Light informs us, space allows the light to shine.

"My spine, moving Like kelp in the ocean's bed."
—Anna Halprin

DEEP SEA DIVING

Imagine you are a deep-sea diver. Your body is made of radiant light and is swimming through newly awakened spaces, unraveling congestion. Your breath is this liquid light, shining radiance into spaces not seen before. The ocean into which you are plunging is the interior of your own body. Dive down toward the perineum, aiming for the center of the small circular area. As you swim through the sea, doing a breaststroke, notice that from that midpoint out to the outer edges of the circle, there are thousands and thousands of reeds that are twisted and torqued and wrapped around each other. With your long arms and fingers, gently move through the congested reeds, between them. They move delicately, separating and providing the spaces for you to swim through. Your limbs are like the exquisite rays of light that you can breathe between the fibers filling the cells with liquid breath, creating more room and more space.

As you swim you may notice areas of congestion, where light is unable to filter through. These places may hold emotional and physical manifestations of that which you have protected yourself from, and wisely so. Notice. Breathe and honor the shadows as much as you honor the spaces. All is here to inform us.

Pain created from holding and protecting may begin to unravel and emotions may arise. Tenderly hold and receive these emerging feelings. This beginning of the unraveling journey has its own timing, its own rhythm. Oftentimes we need support to feel that which is emerging out of the shadows. You may need a friend or a therapist to hold you as you feel these new places.

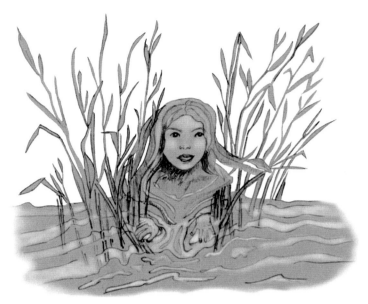

Doing the Breaststroke Through the Reeds

THE FIGURE EIGHT

As you sit and breathe through your perineal body into your chair, remind yourself of the numbers on the clockface. The 3, the 9, the 12 and the 6 are all dropping gently below you, like those long fibers of the sea anemone. Breathe into the circle and imagine it opening wide, so that the one-inch area of the perineum is being breathed into what feels like a two-inch circle.

As we gently open these closed spaces, visualize those back numbers on either side of 6 unraveling and opening like the peacock fanning out its colored feathers behind you. Then the numbers to the left and right of 12 peel open and you are an ever-expanding vessel.

Within this circle, visualize a drawing of a figure eight lying horizontally between 3 and 9. Imagine that this shape is drawn with a pencil of light, so that it glows. Draw the light all around the figure eight starting from the dot in the middle of the perineal body and moving the light up and into and around the upper right quadrant between 12 and 1, passing by 2 and then streaming down past 3 and around to 4 and 5. Between 5 and 6, the light

curves up through the midpoint of the perineal circle (body) and up and
around to the upper left quadrant, between 12 and 11.

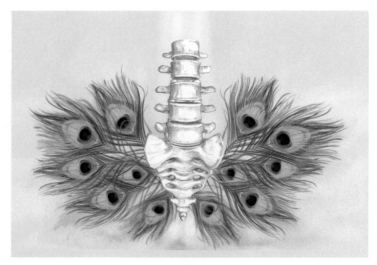

Expanding Wider

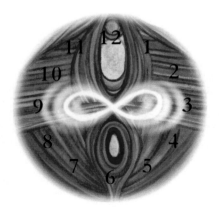

Moving the Light

Move the light slowly with your breath, your inhalations and exhalations
guiding your pace. The light sweeps around all the numbers in the left
quadrants, passes by 10, 9 and 8, and 7. Once again, before reaching 6, it
moves up through the central point into the upper right quadrant, around
the lower right, though the middle again, up into the upper left, and down

into the lower left. The energy moving that light around the perineal body will begin to seep out wider into your entire perineum. Begin feeling that gentle movement softly undulating out of the perineal body into the entire perineum, into the corners of the upper thighs and around behind the sacral bones and in the front behind the pelvic bones, your hip bones.

Sink the front of the perineum through the soft fabric of your seat as if you are seated on the softest of cushions. Gently surrender the abdominals into the back body, filling the inner back wall of your sacrum delicately.

Now begin to move the figure eight even wider, drawing that light closely around the spine from behind the sacrum. Let it move all the way up and around the spine, traveling slowly behind the ribcage, breathing the light wherever you focus your attention.

As you move into the throat and into the neck, from the base of one side of the skull to the other, sweep the light up into the head, between the two hemispheres of the brain. Explore this moving energy and make the eight wider as you travel back down all the way to your seat. You might bring the light all the way into the outer edges of your body, including your hips, which may want to roll around as you move in this figure-eight motion. Allow your whole body to gently explore this movement. Your head will roll around with the flow, and how much you expand will change each time you practice. The movement that began in your perineal body expands, taking your body on an energetic journey.

> *Try to be a sheet of paper with nothing on it.*
> *Be a spot on the ground where nothing is growing.*
> **—Rumi**

You can also practice this visualization while standing. Start from the midpoint in the perineum and begin to allow the light of your drawing to move you gently. Feel your feet expanding into the earth, melding with the earth, growing roots through your feet deeper and deeper. Explore the movement of the light in your ankles, your knees, your hips, around the spine and in your armpits so that your arms and your torso begin to follow the movement of the figure eight like a gentle moving tree being caressed by the wind. The light is moving you. The energy is moving you. You are expanding and widening your structure. Play with the movement that is swinging internally around the bowl of your pelvis. Play and explore with the curiosity of a child.

A SEA SPONGE

Another visual that I resonate with is that of a sea sponge. When you squeeze a sponge and then release it, the holes become wider, so that air can fill every space. Contractions and constrictions created through misalignment suffocate and squeeze the cells, ultimately imprisoning the energy within the cell. These contracted muscle-fiber cells begin to create distorted patterns. They attach to the bones in their distorted manner and literally pull the bones out of alignment. These patterns begin to *in*form us and *re*form us, patterns leading to pain. When we begin to unravel, it is as if we are releasing that sponge, allowing the breath to fill the spaces.

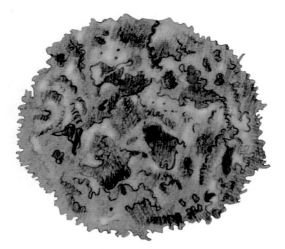

Expanding the Cells with Space

As you practice, play with this image of the sea sponge. Imagine placing it at a particular point in your body, on a tightly wound area that you want to focus on.

As you breathe in fill the sponge with awareness, as if with light.

On the exhales, allow the light to seep out of the cells into the vast space surrounding these cells. Feel the musculature expanding as the cells become bigger spaces to explore. Space provides the opportunity to redesign our musculature. Space allows the cell structure the freedom to realign muscle over bone, bringing so much more information. As muscles move off and over bone, bone can move, and the redesign begins.

THE PARACHUTE

When a parachute begins its descent from the great height above us, the inner dome shape of the silk fills evenly all the way around, like a perfect bowl turned upside down.

As you sit on a chair, envision a tiny parachute sailing down above your head and beginning its descent through your crown. The upper palette in the mouth is shaped exactly like this inner dome of the parachute. The perineum is shaped like an inverted dome. The upper dome and the lower dome would fit together like a globe—one of the many mysteries of our sacred geometry.

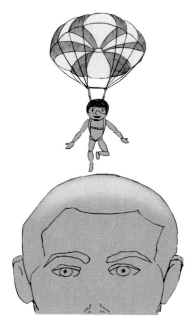

Connecting From Above

Run your tongue on the upper palette all the way around the dome, sweeping way back to where the fibers holding the tongue into the back of the throat are connected. Breathe behind and around these connections.

As this wondrous parachute sails through the spine, through the nervous system, gently quieting you, it moves all the way down through the perineum, the integrity of the silk completely expanded all the way around. As you breathe through the perineum and feel the parachute dropping onto the seat of the chair, the heaviness of your thighs falls deeper. You are now releasing through the center point and as the lines emanating from the central point are smoothed out, you become wider on the seat. The muscle fibers are elongated and gently persuaded to expand. Their hold on the bones releases. Like the parachute sailing to earth, fall tenderly into the fabric of the chair.

This may seem like a funny image, but it's one I have found helpful: imagine the parachute sailing to the earth and picture twelve little people taking hold of the lines, like cords, growing out of the midpoint, gently wiggling the wrinkles completely out of the silk so that when it lands, there is a perfect circle lying on the earth.

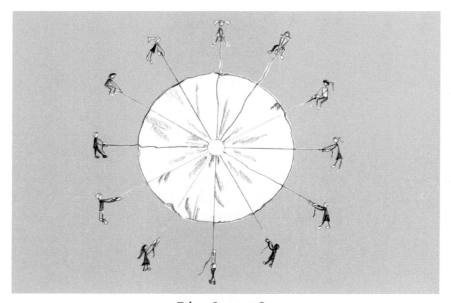

Fibers Ironing Out

Imagine that those strands are emanating from the midpoint of the perineum. They can be breathed open, widening and expanding the pelvis so that you can sit deeper through the base. As you descend deeper, breathing deeply into the spaces, relax the lower torso, drop the heels through the earth and begin to lift the upper torso out of the pelvic floor. Feel the leg bones sliding out of the pelvis, the knees looking forward over the toes, helping the spinal muscles stretch, growing you taller.

THE HANGING SKELETON

One of my clients finds this visualization one of the most helpful. Stand tall, with your sacrum wide and open behind you, the numbers all around the perineum expanding out with those rays of light. The abdominals breathing into the back body, towards your sacrum, allow your sacral muscles to slide off your small sacral bones.

With your heels falling into the earth, imagine there is a hook on the top of your head, and you are hanging from a cord that waves from the crown, through your spine and into the base. You are connected to a pole above you, like a skeleton hanging in an anatomy class.

Allow the breath to wave through your crown and all the way through your pelvic floor. You are weightless and completely supported.

For further resources to support your inquiry, including videos, guided audio exercise, and more visit:

www.corebodywisdom.com

CHAPTER 9

RETURNING TO YOUR ROOTS: VARIATIONS ON THE SQUAT

"To be rooted is perhaps the most important and least recognized need of the human soul."
—Simone Weil

IN THIS CHAPTER and the next, I will suggest various stretches to help you create movement from the base, and unravel the distortion in the perineum. By now you have an idea of the imbalance in the floor of your pelvis, one that has been deeply drawn into the musculature and has literally moved bones out of alignment. As you become more and more aware (within and around the small area of the perineum), the way you move becomes increasingly and vitally important.

The stretches I teach you will create openings and deeper awareness that you can carry with you as you practice other forms of exercise or movement modalities. Any form of movement—whether it be yoga, Pilates, dance, cycling, running, golf, tennis, swimming, or simply walking down the street—provides an opportunity to bring more and more awareness to your pelvic floor, allowing the movement to emerge organically. (I'll be addressing specific types of exercise in chapter 12).

We have lost our center, especially in Western industrialized cultures, and these stretches I present are your way home to that center. Continue to be aware of the collapse into one side of your pelvis and the squeezing of the fibers in and around the perineum, between the sacrum and the coccyx, the fibers tucking the buttocks under so that the tailbone (the coccyx), retreats under and in toward the perineum. Be aware of your numbers! Keep the image of the clockface in your mind as you progress through these exercises.

Male Perineal Clockface

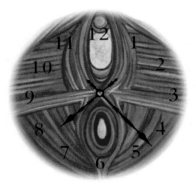

Female Perineal Clockface

Props to have ready:

◆ a folded blanket, low pillow or towel for under your heels
◆ a chair to practice dropping, sitting onto
◆ a counter top, back of the couch, or banister to hold on to as you slowly allow the sacral muscles to release off the bone and toward the floor

Remember, take your time with these exercises and rest as often as you need to. The movements may seem small but the degree of focus is intense. Hold the posture for long enough that it begins to inform you, and remember, you can always come up and out whenever you want to, with awareness coming up as much as descending. Read all the way through the instructions once or twice before you practice, and then refer to them as often as you need.

LIFE AS A SQUAT

The squat is one of the most important postures in SRI because it represents the correct alignment of the spine. Although this may sound strange, when your body is aligned, no matter what position you are in, you are always in a squat. How can it be that while standing, you are in a squat? While sitting in a chair you are in a squat? Let's look more closely, with the help of the world's best squatter, the baby.

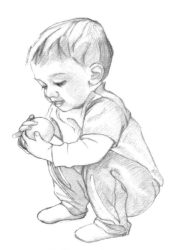

Life as a Squat

If you look at the illustration of the baby in a squat, notice how far back the pelvis is from the heels. The sacrum, the lowest part of the vertebral column with the tail at the base, is very much behind the heels and the heels are dropped into the earth, softly yet firmly. When I squat, I like to imagine that I am performing this stretch in sand and slowly being received into the earth. See how the baby's spine elongates out of the open perineum all the way up through the crown.

STANDING AND SQUATTING

The squat begins in your standing posture. As you stand, can the spine balance precisely through the bony structure with the weight evenly distributed equally on the heels and the ball of the toes? Or, are you falling more into the front of your feet or to the back of the heels? The standing posture practice (Chapter 7) will guide you into all others.

Now, let's begin to move toward a squat. Do not try to get all the way down, but notice when you begin to descend even a few inches how soon your chest leans forward, with your head falling away from the cervical and thoracic vertebrae, your heels lifting up off the floor, your weight moving forward over the toes. Do not hold yourself in the pose; come up again.

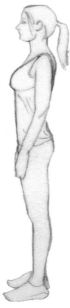

Standing in Anatomical Balance

Now compare what you just did to the baby (see illustration, page 163). As the baby relaxes into the squat, can you see the length, the stretch in the lowest part of the back, the sacrum hanging off the lumbar spine, the lumbar spine hanging off the thoracic and the thoracic hanging off the cervical? The back of the skull is directly in line with the low back, completely in alignment, in "biomechanical tune," to use Beach's terminology. The child can play with objects in front and all around for a long time without losing balance.

Stand upright with your feet a bit wider than hip-width apart (Remember, hip width is determined by drawing a line through the center of the pelvic bones.) For the practice of the squat, you may find that the wider your feet are away from the midline the easier it is to drop down and stay in your heels. Keep the kneecaps soft even before your knees are beginning to bend.

"A silent body is a body that has a natural dignity."
—Dona Holleman

Look into the back of the perineal area with your mind's eye. Open the fibers between 6, 5, 4 in the lower right quadrant and those between 7, 8, 9 in the lower left quadrant. Notice if your feet are falling to the inside arches and open between fibers 12, 1, 2 in the upper right quadrant and those between 12, 11, 10 in the upper left. You can put your thumb of each hand into the root of the thigh and the other fingers lying around the top and along the side of the thigh. Gently, as you breathe and imagine the numbers in the upper quadrants opening, allow your fingers to guide the flesh from the inner thigh out from the midline. Allow the front of the perineum at 12 to look down. As you open the perineum like the petals of a flower, all petals emerging out of the middle of the flower unfurling, feel the fibers of the quadricep muscles lying on the femur bones begin to softly peel away from the center, allowing the inside flesh of the knees to emerge, the kneecaps aligning over the top of the feet. Release the sphincters in the floor of the pelvis, for squeezing will create the same tucked-under feeling that you have probably lived with forever.

With your fingertips resting gently on your upper thighs, apply a little bit of pressure into the muscle, and the femurs will gently recede into the back of your legs, moving you away from your toes and transferring some of the weight into your heels. Your toes may even lift up off the floor. They are free to elongate now. Like stretching your fingers out of the palm of your hand you can crawl the toes out of the back of the arches, feeling a long stretch all the way through your arches. In actuality, you are allowing your toes to emerge from the open perineum, as that is where they originally emerged from. Remember that the limb buds emerge at about six weeks in utero.

Wearing shoes causes the toes to grab the earth under us to walk and I want you to feel the toes having the ability to stretch, elongate all the way out of the back of the arch of the foot. You may even feel tension in the arch because it has been so shortened. We have muscles everywhere and some have not ever been lengthened!

As you walk your toes out, you can feel the base of the toes, especially the ball of the big toe. Toes widening apart, baby toe stretching away from the fourth toe, you are standing wide across the base of the feet, the outer heel planted and the inner heel as well aware of the potential collapse in the arches.

Fanning out the numbers of the perineum allows the leg bones to widen away from the midline and you can feel the widening of the sacral muscles, like a peacock fanning out its feathers.

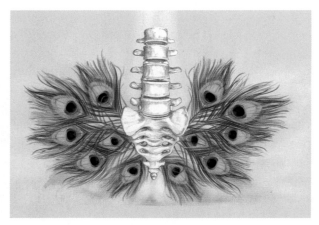

Fanning Out

You may feel like you are falling backwards, your buttocks way back. Remember the image of those mannequin poles that are emerging from that "eye behind the thigh" at the base of the butt. If you gently bring the abdominal muscles behind the pubic bone into the back body toward the sacrum, the muscles of the sacrum will slide off the bones and bring you down into the beginning of the squat, which is the internal feeling we want to recognize even while standing upright. This action will also bring the imaginary mannequin poles down toward the floor, way back behind the heels, like a second pair of legs.

Remember to check and see if you are squeezing the anal muscles to hold you in this new place of alignment. If so, release. Inhale, and on your exhale allow the ribcage to fall. You may now feel as if you are falling backwards and your chest wants to fall forward in reaction. Remember to counter this feeling by engaging your abdominals at the bottom of the pelvis behind your pubic bone. You can gently place your fingertips into the flesh above the pubic bone and apply a gentle pressure. In that space right above the pubic bone, feel the expansion out through the sacrum behind you. Breathe from the middle of the sacrum out to the sides as if the breath, like gentle fingers, spreads the muscle fibers apart, widening your entire base, which also brings the awareness to the outer heels. Elongate your toes out of the back of the arches to distribute the weight more evenly between the balls of the toes and the heels.

Your head has probably fallen forward.

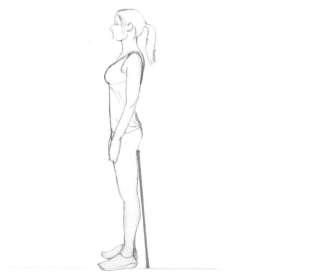 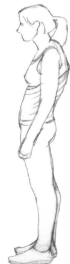

Your Second Pair of Legs   *The Great Collapse*

As you breathe your ribcage down and the muscles under your armpits (the "lats" or *latissimus dorsi*) relax as well, you can imagine the abdominals all the way under your fingertips behind the pubic bone rolling up so that the upper torso lifts out of the pelvis. The crown of your head emerges out of the perineum and stretches all the way up and out of your base as your leg bones climb all the way down out of the pelvis moving deeply through the earth. Stand in your upright posture for several breaths, feeling into your body. You will feel a whole assortment of muscles "talking" to you I am sure! Breathe.

Now you are ready to try a squat again. It is best to come in and out, feeling your way deeper into the openings each time. This is your exploration and any time you need to begin again, give yourself permission to do so. You are reeducating your muscle fibers all the time.

With your fingertips in the root of the thighs (where the femur and the pelvic floor meet) keeping the abdominals in the back body, feel the sacrum beginning to slowly drop down toward and back behind your heels.

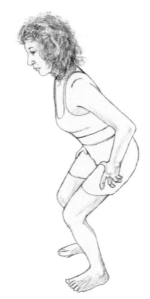

Creating Space

Think of your tailbone pointing backwards and imagine you have a long dinosaur tail unfurling.

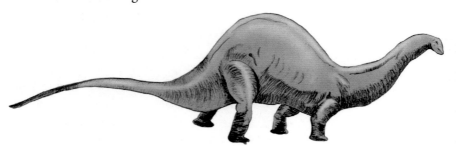

Unfurling Your Tail

Those imaginary mannequin poles fall straight down behind the back of the heels as if you have another pair of feet to stand on. It is the sacral muscles that begin your descent into your squat, and will ask the knees to bend.

With your knees bending, allow the base of the buttocks to move back even more. With all those open numbers around the perineal clockface and with the abdominals gently in the back, allow the pelvis to hang off your upper torso. You do not need to go down very far to feel the sacrum hanging off your thoracic spine (your mid back). Space is created at the waist area and in the lumbar area where the shortening is usually profound. Here is where you hang the pelvis, hang the arms, breathe the ribcage away from your upper chest, and fill the pelvic bowl with breath.

Let your facial muscles release and your tongue hang loosely in your mouth. Remind the abdominals behind the pubic bone to stay in the back toward the sacrum. The sacrum begins to hang even more. The low back will likely feel achy as the muscles elongate, and you will be tempted to rush out of this stretch to escape the intensity. Breathe deeply and come up slowly.

Coming back into an upright posture, grow your leg bones out of the pelvis, extend your feet down as if through soft sand, stretch the leg bones into the earth. Roll the abdominals into the back body, and stand all the way upright. As the legs reach all the way out of the pelvis and your upper torso rises up out of the base, you will begin to feel the stretch of the psoas muscle more and more.

You may feel that stretch all the way up to your mid back as your upper torso emerges higher out of the pelvis. Breathe and sigh.

Pay attention to how you are standing: more in the back of the heels, the base of the butt hanging. If you were to drop down again into a squat the base of the butt would draw straight down in line with those mannequin poles. This is what it means to be standing in a squat. Feel those poles emerging out of the "eyes."

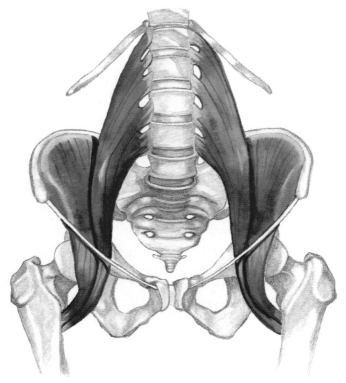

Using Your Psoas to Stand Upright

A DEEPER SQUAT WITH SUPPORT

So let's squat again with some support to allow you to deepen farther down.
Find a countertop, railing, or table where you can gently place your fingers.
Stand perhaps two of your feet lengths away from the counter. You will adjust
this space between your feet and the counter as you practice and open the
base even more. You may find that you need to back farther away the next
time you descend because your weight is no longer on the toes. You may also
want to fold or roll up a towel or a blanket for under your heels. Don't make
it too high, just enough so that as you unravel the sacral muscles you can
comfortably sink your heels into the roll.

As you breathe the ribcage down, flooding the breath like a river of warm
light into the pelvic floor, bring the low abdominals gently toward the back

body, widening and freeing the sacral muscles. Your numbers open and you become aware of particular areas of contraction. Slowly exhaling, let the base of the buttocks open and move back; attend to the back numbers unfurling, the sacral muscles sliding off the bones, taking you toward that squat. Unravel the head up out of the pelvis as every exhalation guides you deeper into your pelvic bowl.

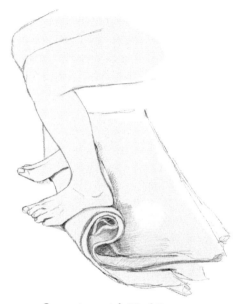

Squatting with Heel Support

As your knees bend and you are gently taken into the squat, envision the front of the perineum at 12 o'clock looking down. Release the buttock muscles so that the breath, the river of warm liquid light, can flow through the center of the perineum.

Feel the ever-expanding pelvic floor, your feet widening as the bones of your legs are not squeezing inward. Breathe, exhale way down into your base. With every exhale, remind the belly muscles behind the pubic bone to retreat quietly into the back body. As you hold on to the table top, drop your shoulders. Drop the ribcage internally, the muscles under your arm pits, and let your shoulder blades slide down your back body. Release all the muscles in your face, including those in your mouth, your tongue, your jaw. Sighing with your out-breaths can be helpful.

Remember, it is the action of keeping the abdominals in the back body that will allow the journey to begin toward this archetypal posture, which lives in our cellular and cultural history. You do know how to do this. You have the information embedded deep within your cells. It is always there. You are freeing up the entanglements that have kept you in the dark, kept you away from your divine birthright.

Slowly begin your descent—receiving it, not demanding it. Gently hold on to the counter top or whatever your hands are using for support, breathe and open all the perineal numbers wider, the fibers expanding out of the middle, look 12 o'clock downwards, and gently move the abdominals behind the pubic bone toward the sacrum. Flood the sacrum and the pelvic bowl with breath, allowing the sacral muscles to peel away from your sacral bone and take you down toward your squat.

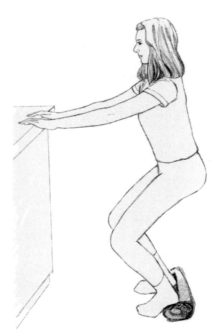

Squatting with Upper Body Support

As you descend you will feel your back numbers tucking under.

Whenever you feel the flesh retreating under, breathe once again into the center of the perineum and fan out all the lines like that starburst of light.

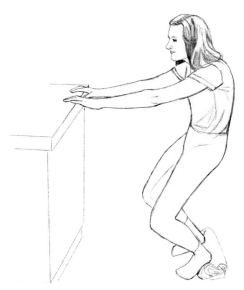

Squatting with Collapsed Spine

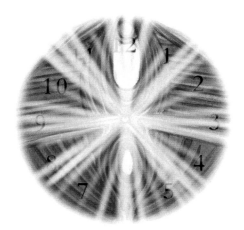

Squatting with the Rays of Light Expanding

Opening the back numbers between the tailbone and the thighs will keep your mannequin poles way back, and the abdominals once again in the back body will keep those poles reaching back and down behind your heels to the ground.

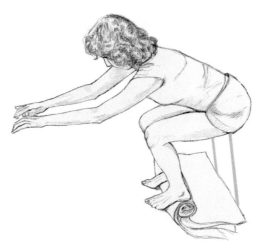

Where Are Your Extra Feet?

As you drop deeper, keep opening and sending your sacrum back so that at the top front of the thighs you are not closing off the space between the pelvis and the thigh. Keep the abdominals in the back body as well. I know this is not an easy feat. The tucking of the pelvis for a whole lifetime pushes the femurs way forward so that we lose space and freedom to move the legs down and out and the spine up and out.

I want to keep reminding you that neurology is not your friend here. We have all informed the brain to believe that the way we have carried our structure is the way it is supposed to be. Now you are *re*informing the neurology and this takes time and practice. Thousands of muscle-fiber cells are being informed and they will notify hundreds of thousands and millions more each time you practice—this I can promise you!

You do not need to go all the way down in your squat. It is more important to follow the alignment and the opening, way back in the sacrum and pelvic floor. As far down as you do go, drop the heels through the folded blanket. Using your hands on the counter, railing, or table, you can monitor how much you can move downwards and breathe through the open pelvic floor. Your femur bones are heavily received into the back of your legs and the base of the butt (the "eyes") moves back toward your heels. The front of the perineum (12 o'clock) looks down. Keep reminding yourself to notice where the skull is. Unwind it out of the pelvis so that you are not hanging the heavy weight of the head forward. The sacrum is your guide.

If you do go all the way down into your full squat, keep deepening the heels and filling the pelvis, breathing between the sacral bones and the musculature covering those little bones. We can get movement in between the tiny bones in the sacrum, the spaces where we once had cartilage (usually by the age of eighteen, the cartilage is gone and these bones are said to be fused together, but we do have the memory of the space between the bones). With correct alignment, the spinal muscles alongside the sacral bones can stretch and create space.

"In order to change our body shape or our movement patterns we must change our neurological activity."
—Irene Dowd

When you are ready to come up from your squat, keep the breath moving downwards through your torso into the bowl, into the base, and sink those heels deep into your rolled blanket as the bones in your legs straighten while the heels descend through the blanket. Lift your upper torso up out of your pelvis, and watch for that tucking of the tail. On the way up, you may need to stop and say, "Where is my butt? Where are those mannequin poles? Did they just retreat under?" Open the numbers.

You will quite likely feel a desire to rise quickly. Coming through this space is difficult, even painful, because your body is using muscles it never knew existed! You are now engaging your inner thighs (the adductors) and the psoas to support your ascent. Even when you feel that your legs are perfectly straight, you can still crawl them further out of your pelvis and bear the weight into the earth.

Again, the squat is always present in a full standing posture. Remember the mannequin poles emanating from the base of the butt ("eyes behind the thighs") down and through the earth. Unwinding your upper torso out of the base as the legs go deeper and deeper, you create more room for the poles to be those extra pair of legs to stand on. Stretching the leg bones allows the back muscles to make room between vertebrae, which in turn provides more room to enliven the discs in between. Spaciousness is what you want to create, to feel what has been hidden deep within the tissues of the body.

If you can devote fifteen minutes a day, twice daily, to practicing your squat, you will see amazing results. You might, after a while, be able to drop down into your squat without the use of a counter top.

You may also find that releasing into what is such a magical posture begins to inform you in many ways, opening up pathways for energy to flow more freely.

Remember, this was a basic posture we all spent much time in, deep in our evolutionary past. Your neurology may be surprised to meet those emotional places that have perhaps been hidden in the past, awakening you, informing you. Make space for the light to *in*form. Evolution is always happening.

CHAIR SQUAT

This exercise is similar to the sitting exercise I shared in Chapter 7, but now that you have practiced the squat, you may recognize more deeply how your seated posture is, in fact, the posture of the squat.

Sitting on a chair, close to the front of the seat, with your lower legs perpendicular to your thigh bones, once again feel the feet on the floor.

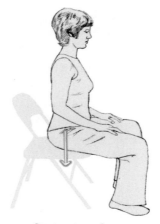

Sitting in a Squat

If the heels drop into the earth below the floor you are in essence standing on your feet exactly the same as if you are standing upright. When the heels drop through the earth your spine automatically rises up out of the pelvic floor when your pelvic floor is in the anatomically correct position.

As you sit forward towards the lip of the seat, drop the front of the perineum at 12 o'clock forward and down onto the lip of the chair seat.

With your fingertips underneath your buttocks, very close to the inner corners where the femur comes into the base of the buttocks, stretch the flesh so that your back numbers open. As you open the right side first, feel the stretch of 3 o'clock across the perineal body. You might feel as if you are seated deeper into that right side. Breathe and notice the difference between the two sides. Perhaps the left fibers from 9 o'clock to the midpoint of the imaginary clockface feel as if they are shortened or folded into the midpoint. Open the left.

You may go back and forth to each side as more fibers give way so that you can be sitting more directly on that dot in the middle of the perineal body clockface.

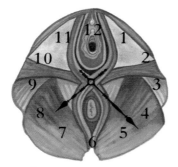

"One" With the Chair

If you remember the image of the swimmer in Chapter 8, you are providing a wider and more open base, detangling the fibers that are twisted on, around, and under each other so that the swimmer can pass through. As your arms open the fibers, separating them like reeds in the sea, you have a lot more room to create an open pathway; the area between the sacrum and coccyx (the very base of the spine) is spread wide.

With the area around the whole perineum open, 12 o'clock can breathe deeply down into the chair seat. If you are sitting on a softer cushion, let go of the sphincters and feel the center of the perineum melt through the cushion, the energy flowing all the way down through the earth. In essence, you are not seated on the chair but through the chair.

With the abdominals breathing gently toward the back body, behind the sacrum, 6 o'clock drops down into the cushion as well. Widen your whole circle in every direction flooding the center out to all the lines with your breath. Like a starburst, or fireworks opening in a most colorful array from the midpoint all the way out, feel the expansion of your entire base. Just as in your standing posture, the sacrum widens because you have put the pelvis in anatomical position and you can now roll the abdominals up toward the upper chest. Your upper torso is rising out of the base and your lower torso is releasing heavy through the seat of the chair.

Now, you are squatting on the chair. Notice how similar this posture is to the standing squat. Your thighs and pelvis are so heavy that if the chair was removed you would deepen all the way down to the floor. Continue to melt through the chair, because shortly you are going to emerge up out of the seat, leaving the weight of the pelvis hanging as your legs straighten down through the floor out of the pelvis.

MOVING UP FROM THE CHAIR
AND BACK DOWN

Now the fun begins. You are going to get up out of your chair and descend back into it. I like to think of this exercise as the "Walker Prevention Stretch" because it requires that you stand evenly in your leg bones, developing the strength that will keep you on your own two feet for many decades to come.

Sit in your chair. You may want to put another chair directly in front of you for balance, facing you, about 1.5 to 2 feet away, as if you were about to have a conversation with its occupant. However, if you use a chair this way your hands should be barely touching it. The weight of the upper torso is not hanging forward onto the front chair as you would if you had a walker directly in front of you to help you ascend.

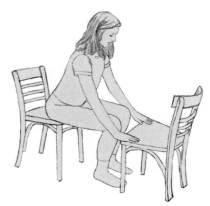

Readying to Stand in Your Squat

Once again, release 12 o'clock to look down, move the abdominals back, open the back numbers, and sink deeper through the seat as you elongate your upper torso.

Unscrew your spine and your skull higher and higher out of the descending heavy pelvis. Breathe your ribcage internally down, filling the back body behind the lumbar region and the sacral bones with breath. Do this several times.

Let 12 o'clock tip farther forward so that your upper torso is leaning at an angle and place your fingertips on the lip of the seat of the chair in front of you. The arm bones now have space to elongate out of the pelvis, taking your hands farther onto the seat. Keep the belly in the back so that the sacrum is still hanging and you are still climbing your head up and out of the base, instead of rounding your whole upper torso forward. Make sure your back numbers and the flesh under the thighs have not receded back into your pelvic floor. You may need to use your fingers again to stretch them wide open.

Your lower legs are perpendicular to your thighs and your feet are straight.

Moving the feet down through the floor, raise your pelvis off the chair just a few inches and keep hanging the pelvis as if you are going to sit back on the chair, as in your squat.

Breathe the ribcage down, flood the bowl with breath, look 12 o'clock down toward the chair. Holding your belly muscles behind the pubic bone in the back keeps 6 o'clock moving down.

Hang the center of the circle back and down toward the chair.

Slowly release back onto the chair, allowing the perineum to descend through the chair!

Take some breaths here and enjoy the sitting and stretching of the sacrum, growing your upper torso up, out, and off your thighs. Keep your upper body growing out of the perineum, the crown of your head emerging out of the hanging perineum.

Now let's climb all the way to standing, always hanging the base toward the chair to keep stretching those sacral muscles. Place your hands lightly, if you like, on the seat of the other chair in front of you.

The heavy head will always want to fall forward. Roll the head up so that the back of the skull aligns with the base of the spine.

Ready for lift off? With your feet pressing through the floor, begin to lift off the chair . . . slowly . . . slowly. Move your leg bones longer and longer through the floor, stretching them out of the pelvis, as if you are growing them down and into the earth like roots. As they straighten you are breathing into the back body, elongating the sacrum.

As you stand on your feet, your legs keep unwinding through the ground, move the abdominals back and undulate the upper torso out of the base.

Feel the separation between the top of your thighs and the very bottom of the pelvic bones. If you put your fingertips in that space, you can wiggle yourself up and out even more. It feels like rolling the belly muscles up off your legs.

Notice if your numbers at 6, 5, and 4, and 6, 7, and 8 have started to retreat. Of course they did! Once again, open the back of the perineum, which will stretch the flesh under the upper thighs toward the chair behind you.

With the "belly in the back," once again you will feel the abdominals lengthening the sacral muscles and naturally you will begin to make your way back down to the chair behind you.

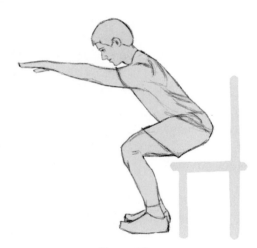

Almost There

Notice that if you were to tuck the butt under, you would miss the chair altogether! You want the "eyes behind the thighs" to land on the chair first.

The chair is going to seem like it is a mile underneath you. Slowly breath your way all the way back onto the seat—this is much harder than simply plopping down. Feel the stretch of the sacral muscles and the abdominals. If you feel like you are going to lose balance, you can use your fingers to find the seat behind you.

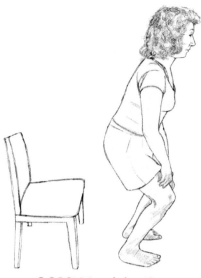

OOPS! Missed the Chair

Practice the sitting and standing two to three times and take a break. Have fun with this, and take your time. It is not easy.

WELL-DESERVED RELAXATION

Periods of relaxation are as important as the periods of activity. When you stretch, you are providing the map, the path to help your system orient to a new structure. It is in the relaxation of the muscle fibers that the cells actually learn the new way of alignment—which is actually not new at all, but embedded in our neurology, deep in our ancestral heritage. Creating space allows ancient wisdom to come forth and inform you. Relaxation allows the system to orient to the new structure. It is in stillness that we learn how the new way of stretching has informed our structure.

Let's return to the lying down pose we practiced in Chapter 7. You will now be coming into this pose with more information and awareness than you had when we began.

Lay down on your back, with knees bent and feet on the floor. If you need a blanket roll to place under the back of the knees, have one available—I will indicate when it is time to place it.

The Achilles tendons should be aligned with the base of the butt, the "eyes behind the thighs." Place your elbows on the floor close to your torso. Put weight through the floor with your elbows. Breathe your ribcage down and fill your back body with breath. Then elongate your spine out of the base by crawling your upper back, one shoulder at a time, out of your pelvis. You can then put your fingertips on your pubic bone and stretch the flesh away through the legs so that you have more space available to once again crawl your upper torso away. Release the 12 o'clock point on the perineal circle to gently look down between your legs. The abdominals fall into the back body with gravity. Begin to elongate one leg with the heel stretching out of the perineum, rolling the bones in the leg in and out, so that you feel as if the leg bone is unscrewing longer and longer from behind the musculature. Elongate your other leg the same way. Feel the psoas muscle extending the leg all the way out from the pelvic bones and the connection with the muscles on either side of the spinal column in the lumbar region. Remember, this is where the psoas connects the spine with the pelvis, with the legs. (Sing the children's song, "the knee bone's connected to the thigh bone," just for fun!).

Again, with your elbows on the floor close to your upper torso, lower arms bent and fingers pointed up to the ceiling, put weight on your elbows and crawl your upper body longer and longer in the opposite direction of your legs. Make sure your ribs are breathing down toward your pelvis and you are filling the lumbar area with breath, exactly as you do when standing.

If you need the blanket roll under your knees to help you drop the sacrum, buttocks, and legs deeper into the floor, place that now.

Release your arms to your sides and relax your legs, letting the feet and thighs roll open as they want to.

Breathe the ribcage internally down, hang the pelvis, hang the sacrum, the entire back body, as if in the hammock of your own back body, and breathe into the floor, through the floor.

Stay here as long as it feels good. Ten minutes of relaxation provides the muscle fibers with the information they need as to what just happened. The muscle-fiber cells become intelligent and receive the realignment of your musculature as they are at rest. In the stillness, movement is happening and your neurology becomes rewired with the new movement patterns.

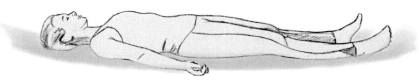

Merging With Your Hammock

CLIMBING THE WALL!

If you keep the experience of your squat in your mind and body, then you can begin to practice putting your spine into extension in other stretches that will deepen your understanding and create more and more space between the vertebrae of the spinal column. The chair pose will continually inform your musculature as you move into these more advanced poses.

Stand in front of a wall with your feet approximately two of your own feet lengths away from the wall. In your standing posture, with your "eyes-behind-your-thighs" and all of your perineal numbers flowering open, allow your heels to gently drop into the floor. Unscrewing the leg bones out of the pelvis, breathe the ribcage down and fill your back body and the pelvis with breath as if you are pouring a warm river down the length of the spine. You should feel the same relaxation that you feel lying down, although it is more challenging because you are weight-bearing.

Start bringing your arm bones up and place your fingertips on the wall the height of your shoulders, shoulder-width apart. That means that the space in between your index and middle fingers is in line with the crease where the upper arm bone (the humerus) meets the armpit corner. Do not lean on the wall, or press into the wall. You want your weight down through the legs and your sacrum, which should be full and expanded, ready to drop down onto a chair as if there were one just inches behind you. If you lean on the wall then your head will fall forward and your chest as well.

With your fingertips barely touching, focus on your back body, focus on that river flowing. Your abdominals should be in the back body toward the sacrum, and 12 o'clock in your perineal body should be facing down. Your head will want to fall forward, but should this happen you would not have your crown circle aligned with your perineal circle. As the chest is brought away from the wall the back of the neck (the cervical spine) has the possibility of coming into alignment with the base of the spine. Breathe the shoulders down away from the ears, allowing your shoulder blades to glide down the back body. Breathe . . . breathe . . . breathe.

As you maintain the intention for the sacral muscles to slide off the sacral bones, providing more and more space for the abdominal muscles to unfurl out of the pelvic floor, you create the space needed for the leg bones to crawl through the softer musculature on the leg bones and deeper into the earth.

Begin crawling the fingertips just a few inches up the wall out of the space you have created between the femur bones and the bottom of the pelvic floor. Notice if your shoulders are lifting up towards your ears causing the deltoid muscles on the upper arms to roll inward around the upper arm bones. Probably so. Breathe, relax the shoulders, and concentrate on the lengthening of the sacral area sliding downwards towards that imaginary chair.

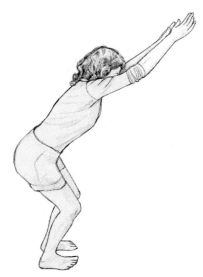

Climbing the Wall

Notice whether the numbers at 6, 5, and 4, and 6, 7, and 8 are retreating and sphincters are squeezing. Remember the peacock feathers fanning.

The wider the two sides of the sacrum expand the more space you have to unscrew the fingers, the arms, and the leg bones out of the pelvic floor.

Breathe the ribcage down. With the lat muscles (on the sides of your torso, under the armpits) breathing down, keep elongating your leg bones out from the pelvis and crawl the fingertips up the wall an inch more, feeling the stretch coming out of your pelvis.

Feel the beginning of the squat, as your knees bend with the relaxing sacral muscles. As your sacral muscles peel off the sacral bones and you feel the beginning of a descent, keep the fingertips exactly where they are on the wall. They will want to slide down as you are internally feeling that squat towards the chair. If anything, climb them up a bit higher and feel that stretch in the whole length of your back.

It is not important how high you are crawling up the wall, a few inches may be the most intense workout if you are aware of your low back descending, belly in the back so that 6 o'clock descends and 12 o'clock looks down as well.

Consistently monitor where your head has migrated to, when your upper chest has fallen forward. Moving your structure minimally brings your awareness into those specific places along the spine that are resistant to stretch. The space you are creating in the low lumbar spine and sacral region is saving your discs and growing you taller!

WALL STRETCH

Let's build this previous stretch into what in yoga is termed a wall stretch.

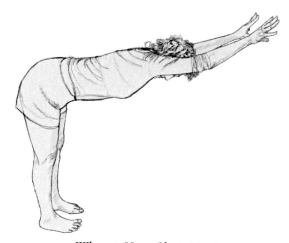

Where is Your Chair Now?

Your intention with this stretch is to increase the space between the upper torso and the lower, between the vertebrae in the lower back (the lumbar) and the sacrum.

Remember how your "climbing the wall" stretch felt. Recall the posture of the squat, which is indelibly written in your being. To begin with, start with your feet the same distance away from the wall as with the previous stretch. Now, slide the hands lower down the wall so that the fingertips are just a bit higher than the eyes (the eyes in your head this time). As you slide your hands down, you will need to walk your feet farther back, one foot length more. Keep the back of the head and the neck in line with the tailbone. Having the chin slightly down elongates the back of the neck.

Gravity is *not* your friend here. Your head is so heavy it will want to collapse toward the floor, as will your chest, causing those upper arm muscles (the deltoids) to collapse inward, squeezing off the space between your inner shoulder and neck. As you lift the chest up away from the floor and the back of the neck as well, the deltoids have more freedom to roll open and around your upper arm bones away from the neck, creating space across your upper back.

"The Light has a request: It asks that you enjoy the process. Connecting to the Light is like taking part in a movie that is guaranteed to have a happy ending."

—Yehuda Berg

Lift the lower ribs that want to collapse to the floor up a little bit into the back body. This helps the upper torso from falling through your inner arms toward the floor. You may feel as if the upper back is rounded like an angry cat, which is exactly the feeling you want. Send your breath all the way down into the pelvis.

The back of your neck stays in line with your low back. This is challenging. Just as in your standing upright posture, where the head tends to fall forward, and the chest to collapse, this stretch is no easier. In fact, it is even more difficult because, as I said, gravity is not your friend!

Keep your kneecaps soft, creating the space between the patella bone and the capsule behind it, instead of hyperextending them and pushing them backwards into the capsule. The muscles on the inner legs and outer legs, alongside the caps, can only stretch if there is space for them to do so. If you need to bend the knees a little more, then do so.

Breathe the river of breath towards the pelvic floor, filling the back body.

Lift the bottom of the abdominals up into the sacral area so that the sacral muscles can elongate away from your lumbar region. Remember, the intention is to create space in the lumbar region where most of the disc problems occur. As you breathe and fill, you will feel the low back and pelvis sliding back away into the room behind you and your weight will now fall solely into the heel bones. This is the indication that you have to walk your feet farther back. Try stepping back one-foot-length more. Ultimately, you will walk back incrementally until your legs are perpendicular to your upper torso. As the spinal muscles on either side of the vertebrae (the erector spinae) elongate the back body, the sacrum is farther back, and that informs you that it is time to step farther back. It does not matter if you get into the completed wall stretch, the right angle pose, as long as you can feel the space in your low back increasing bit by bit. It feels like an ache as the muscles stretch.

Always keep in mind that the eyes behind the thighs are open and if you were to begin sitting down on a chair (see image on page 180) you would want the eyes to lead the way. You can try this, moving toward the chair pose no more than an inch. Keep the belly behind the pubic bones lifted. Open all your numbers. Looking 12 o'clock down, with the abdominals up in the back body, you will begin to experience a deep stretch in between the lumbar and sacrum. If you don't feel it right away, you will eventually.

If you are a practitioner of yoga, you may have done a similar stretch. However, I've seen experienced practitioners of yoga do a wall stretch with their entire upper torso collapsed. Consider also that the popular pose "downward-facing dog" is actually the same pose on a more intense angle, making it more likely that the whole upper chest wants to fall toward your legs.

BATHROOM OPPORTUNITIES!

Why do you think that in other parts of the world, people squat for elimination?

Going to the bathroom—something you do every day—is an excellent opportunity to feel the center of the perineum expanding out to the sides and all around the clock. As you sit on the toilet seat, notice what parts of the underneath thighs are touching the seat and what parts aren't. Which thigh is sitting more on the seat? If you were to release the center of the perineum down into the toilet and continue to expand all the numbers around, what would change? As 12 o'clock looks down and the "belly-in the back" creates the ability for 6 o'clock to drop, the sacral muscles elongate. Breathe the ribcage downward, and let the river of breath flow through the center, truly flow!

Every time I sit, I can now feel that my 6, 5, and 4 (my droopy side) are curled under me toward the center of my perineum. On the seat of the toilet it is even more noticeable because there is all the empty space in between 3 and 9. With your fingertips, you can expand the flesh from the center between 6 and 5 and between 6 and 7. Notice how easily the fabric of the musculature creeps back under.

Now that you are beginning to understand the importance of the squat, you will carry this awareness with you into the next set of exercises designed to lengthen your spine.

For further resources to support your inquiry, including videos, guided audio exercise, and more visit:

www.corebodywisdom.com

CHAPTER 10

DIVING DEEPER: EXTENSIONS FOR THE SPINE

"An innocent body is a body which is balanced only on the bones"
—Dona Holleman

ARE YOU READY to try some new postures? If you're a yoga practitioner, some of these may be familiar to you, but follow the instructions closely— what's different here is that I am guiding you into these postures from the inside out. Too often, in yoga, we impose the poses onto our distorted structure, rather than unraveling the distortion at its source, in the perineum, and allowing the postures to emerge out of that inner realignment.

LYING DOWN: FURTHER EXTENSION

For this stretch, you will need something to hold—a yoga block or a book or a rolling pin will do, anything you can hold onto with both hands. Lie on the floor, the same way you did for the relaxation pose (p. 183)—knees bent, extending your upper torso out of your pelvis and extending your legs one at a time like those giant screws as you breathe the river of your divine breath into your pelvic floor. (You can also do this stretch keeping your knees bent, feet on the floor, the entire time, if this makes it easier for you to keep the base of the sacrum on the floor.)

Keep your leg bones extending, crawling out more and more, and sink the base of your buttocks, your "eyes behind the thighs," and your sacrum. Holding the object, lift your arms toward the ceiling, until they are perpendicular to the body. Breathe the ribcage downwards once again and drop the sacrum deeper into the imaginary hammock of your back body. Notice if you are squeezing the anal sphincter, your butt muscles, and/or your jaw, or if your shoulders are creeping up to your ears. As you breathe, drop the shoulder blades underneath you into the hammock. Allow the shoulders to fall away from the ears. *Relax.*

Now you are ready to climb the object—the book, block, or rolling pin—out of your pelvic floor over the head.

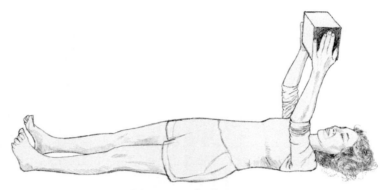

Moving with Alignment

Be aware that as you stretch the arms with the object, your ribcage will likely pop up to your chest and toward the ceiling, creating a bigger curve (lordosis) in your lumbar spinal area. Even taking your arms a few inches closer to your head with the ribcage releasing downward is a huge practice. If you were standing upright and lifting the object up, you would be in the same dilemma with your ribcage, but the dilemma is even more evident lying down. The floor doesn't lie. You will get information if your back body elevates off the imaginary hammock of your musculature. As you feel the rise of the ribcage and the deeper curve in the low back, breathe your ribs toward the pelvic floor, which allows you to receive your breath into that arch. Drop the shoulders away from your ears and the shoulder blades slide down your back. Breathe your entire back body into the support below you.

Keeping everything soft, you may move the arm bones further over your head, however, this may only be inches. As you travel the arms and object overhead more, notice what happens in the sacrum. Did the base of the buttocks lift up? Did the ribcage lift up off your back body? Of course. So, bring your arms back in the opposite direction and lift the object up towards the ceiling bit by bit and see where you can keep falling into the net of support underneath you, for this is when you get the most stretch in the lumbar spine and can crawl the upper torso with the block out even more.

Such a challenge, crawling the leg bones down and out while climbing the upper torso up and out without squeezing your butt or tucking the tail under with all your numbers retreating for dear life! On the floor it is easier to notice, albeit hard to do.

I applaud you for exploring. There is no "wrong" in this practice. Your structure has developed in the way it developed. You might be a world-class athlete with as much distortion as the rest of us. We are all in the same boat of twisted and torqued muscles.

DIVING INTO A FORWARD BEND

Here is an image for you: With your toes hanging off the edge of a diving board and the balls of your toes deeply connected into the board, you are going to roll your upper torso down into a forward bend, falling off the edge into a pool.

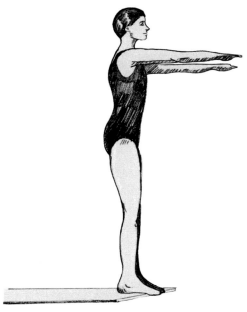

Diving In!

The journey into the water is a long one, for you are really diving into your pelvis, the crown of your head rolling down into your pelvis, creating space between each vertebra as you go. As your head descends, the spine is stretching, even though you are looking completely rounded. You will not jump off the board, you will gracefully fall into your body and roll into the pool.

You already know so much about the position of your body. Standing in an upright posture, imagine you are on the edge of the diving board, and feel the heels descend through the board as if it were made of putty and you are molding into it, the balls of your toes as well. Where is your pelvic floor? Certainly not tucked under with your clockface numbers tucked under your buttock cheeks! Moving the abdominals toward the back body from behind the pubic bone into the sacral wall, keeps the mannequin poles drawing down and back behind the heels, supporting you to stand on the board. You are truly going to need these back legs or a belly flop is imminent!

As you breathe the ribcage down (open all those numbers in the perineal clockface), drop the chin towards your chest and begin rolling your head slowly down, feeling each of the cervical vertebra, one at a time, stretching the spinal muscles alongside. Keeping your shoulders down away from the ears, feel your neck loosen so that the head is just a dead weight and you are not holding it up at all. As you descend into the forward fold, gently bring the abdominals up toward the back body and as you roll down, the abdominals gently undulate upwards through your upper torso. Stretch your sacral muscles off your lumbar spine, lifting the abdominals off the floor of the pelvis, your body extends deeper and deeper over your legs. Continue elongating the sacral area down away from the lumbar and sinking into the board with heels and balls of toes firmly planted.

As you continue to roll, the crown will be facing toward the water and you will begin to offer your head to the pool, while the spinal muscles are extending and stretching you out of your base.

As you roll forward, don't forget your inner squat. It's pretty hard to sit in the squat as you are about to roll into the pool. However, those "eyes behind the thighs" are providing the ballast for this diving body. Remember, you are always stretching in two directions. The mannequin poles are descending down into the board behind you and the upper torso is rolling up and out of the pelvis over your legs. This is exactly the same as in your complete upright standing position.

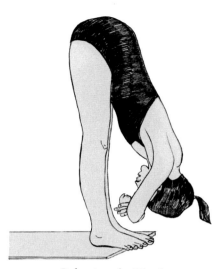

Releasing the Head

Now, you are ready to stand. The "eyes behind the thighs" open, the flower of the perineum open, you are ready for emergence again. Abdominals, where are you? Remind them to stay lifted in the back body.

Slowly begin the journey back up, rolling with focus and intention one vertebra at a time. Breathe the exhalations into the pelvic bowl as you surrender into the base so that as you roll up, you are not lifting out of your base. The base stays full and open and the spinal muscles roll up the side walls of the vertebral column, extending you taller and taller.

When you are three quarters of the way to standing, pause and recheck your pelvis for those retreating numbers. The open numbers and open spaces allow you to crawl those leg bones out and into the diving board, through the board, while you climb your upper torso higher out of the pelvis.

Once you come to standing, breathe deeply and begin the forward roll again. Slowly breathe in between each and every vertebra as you go up and down. *Slow, slow, slow.*

THE CHILD'S POSE

You may be familiar with the yoga pose known as *child's pose*. Let's try this pose with the same awareness we've been bringing to the other stretches.

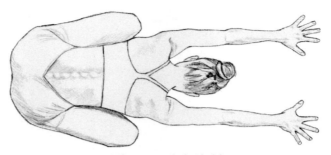

The Extended Child

On all fours, your hands underneath the shoulders and your knees under your upper torso or out to the side of your hips as you see in this illustration, open all around the perineal clock and bring 12 o'clock toward your feet. Remember, we always want the perineal circle to be aligned with the crown circle. Abdominals are up in the back body, and you are breathing the ribcage toward the pelvis.

As you fill the lumbar and sacrum with breath, the sacral muscles begin to elongate your low back and move the "eyes behind the thighs" toward your heels.

If you experience knee pain as you are moving back, you may need to roll up two washcloths and place them securely behind the back of the knees to provide space. The ability to have the base of the buttocks go all the way back on to the heels is a long journey.

As your sacrum extends back, begin walking your hands forward, keeping the back of your neck in line with your tailbone.

Breathe open all the numbers and as your sacrum fills with breath and moves farther back toward the heels, begin to allow your upper torso to round over your thighs (be careful not to tuck those back numbers under). Roll down until you feel the eyes under the thighs dropping closer to your heels while the sacral area stretches open and back, as in the wall stretch. You can now elongate the arms out of your base with the breath, the spinal muscles extending.

For ease and to feel the power of this pose, rest your head on that yoga block or rolled towel so that your head doesn't drop all the way, causing your butt to lift. The stretch is always felt in two directions.

Now, lift the upper torso off your thighs, and away from the floor, keeping the abdominals and the lower ribcage up in the back, so that you have space between the root of the thighs and the bottom of the pelvis, just as in your standing posture. It is all the same pose. The extension of the spine out of the pelvis is always the intention. The "eyes" are dropping down and back behind the heels as your upper thighs descend on to the calves.

You may get tired of me saying this, however it is true: Life is a squat!

SITTING WITH LEGS STRAIGHT OUT AHEAD (DANDASANA)

The preparation for this stretch is no different than sitting on a chair or in your car. Sit down on the floor and put your back body against the wall, bringing the sacrum all the way back into the baseboard. With your finger-tips underneath your thighs, all the way to the space where the inner legs and the bottom of the buttock meet, you can open the back numbers, stretching the flesh on the diagonal out of the center of the perineum toward the wall. The tailbone (the coccyx), has been trained to stay tucked under. Consistent opening between the coccyx and the bottom of the sacrum is always the routine.

Open your legs a foot or two apart, and drop the front of the perineum down toward the floor between your legs.

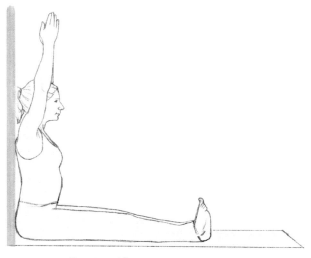

Putting Alignment into Practice

The idea is to create space between the pelvic floor and the legs so that the legs are free to emanate out like those screws, and the pelvis can move independently of the legs. However, you might feel that the legs just want to retreat up into your body because of the lack of space in the root of the thighs (where the femur and the pelvic floor meet).

Place your fingertips on the floor in front of you and drop the front of the perineum into the floor. When the abdominals are in the back body you will feel your sacrum staying in contact with the wall behind you and the back of the perineum (6) rooted. Breathe into your perineum, expanding that one-inch circle, and the thigh bones will be received deeper into the floor. Lift your upper torso out of the base, elongating your spinal muscles, and extend your heels, elongating your legs farther out of the pelvis. If the buttock muscles slide under and forward with your legs, you will need to reach under and open the flesh underneath your thighs once again so those back numbers splay open and your perineum stays wide.

Now, let's try a version of this stretch with a prop. Move away from the wall, fold a blanket so that it is 1 to 1.5 inches thick. Sit on the blanket so that the front of the perineum can land on the front edge and 12 o'clock can drop deeper into the very front edge of the blanket as if it is about to fall off onto the floor. Open the back corners with your fingers once again. You want the feeling of the entire base of the pelvic floor on the blanket. If you draw an imaginary circle on the blanket the perineum would be completely in line with that circle and your spine has room to wiggle up and out.

"Life is movement."

—Bruce Lipton

Breathe the ribcage down and pour the breath, like that river, all the way into the base, the floor of the pelvis. Sink the thighs heavily, especially "the eyes behind the thighs."

You can build on this pose to begin another forward bend, this time in the seated position. Bring your feet closer together, perhaps just a few inches apart. In yoga we are often asked to take a belt around the balls of the feet as we ready for seated forward bend. If you use a belt, hold it very lightly; the balls of the toes should extend the belt away from your body, elongating your legs out of the pelvic floor. Dropping the thigh bones into the floor heavily, especially at the base of the buttocks, will make more room to crawl the legs out of the open perineum.

BOUND ANGLE POSE (BADHA KONASANA)

Another common yoga pose is known as "bound angle." It involves sitting with the knees bent and the soles of the feet together.

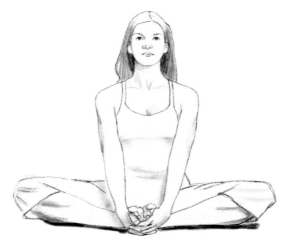

Making Space for 12 to Drop

In this pose, again, it is so difficult to bring the front of the perineum forward and down toward the floor because of the lack of space between the upper leg and the bottom of the pelvis (the root of the thigh). However, as you practice all the other openings, you will create more space in your pelvic floor for the legs to emerge.

Begin as you did for the previous pose. You can bring your low back as close to the wall as you can, opening all the numbers and feeling the difference between the openings in each side.

Bend your knees and bring them toward your pelvis, allowing them to open and bringing the soles of your feet together. You do not have to have the heels all the way into the pubic bone as that makes it much harder to drop 12 o'clock toward the floor. Allow the feet to be a good foot or more away from your pubis—whatever it takes to relax the musculature under the thighs so that you can feel the flesh on the under-thighs in contact with the floor. Breathe deeply into the space between the thigh bone and the bottom of the pelvis, as if you can slide that breath all the way through the quadriceps and bone and through the muscle under the thighs and into the earth.

This stretch can also be done away from the wall seated on a blanket so that the front of the perineum can drop even more. If you have tension in your knees, always move your feet away from the pubis a little more. If you are experiencing knee pain, you can also place a rolled blanket or towel under the thighs closer toward the knee.

As you practice this pose, there is no need to do more than notice the retreating of the back numbers and continue to open those spaces with your intention, your fingers, and your breath.

RELAX!

As always, end your practice sessions lying down and relaxing. If you can plan even five minutes of surrender to allow for the reorganization of cellular wisdom to inform you, realign you, and *re*mind your neurology, transformative healing happens.

Practicing these fundamental postures, with a pelvis in alignment, will bring you back home into your base. The nervous system *re*informs your neurology. The past is never far behind. It is always included in the memory banks of your cellular structure. Time to cash in on the memories! As you are practicing stretches, you are a moving emergence. Behind the distortions and confusions, who are you? This journey of opening and expanding is a mystical experiment.

For further resources to support your inquiry, including videos, guided audio exercise, and more visit:

www.corebodywisdom.com

CHAPTER 11

RE-LEARNING TO WALK: STEP BY STEP

"Healing is the restoration of movement."
—Thomas Hübl

STANDING. SITTING. SQUATTING. Lying down. So far, we've focused on poses that involve little if any movement and yet you are probably amazed by how much goes on in each of these positions. Even being still, in correct alignment, is hard work! And if it takes so much awareness and energy to stay aligned when motionless, what will it mean to do so while in motion? In this chapter, we'll explore one of the most basic forms of movement that you perform every day—walking—and apply the same principles of awareness and alignment that we have learned so far.

Perhaps now, having begun to work with your own realignment, you can share the amazement I felt upon seeing the Masai with such refined dignity moving regally upon the earth.

They maintained alignment effortlessly—legs streaming out of a pelvis seemingly elongating forever, merging deeply into the layers below their feet. They weren't walking on the earth, they were walking through the earth. They belonged to the earth. For the first time I felt I was witnessing the presence of oneness between human and earth. They knew, through their innate body wisdom, a connection to source that informed every movement. I found myself wondering what it would feel like to be so connected, to move so freely. It made me long to feel that depth of relationship with the earth within me. More understanding, more connection, more energy moving through my structure, presencing more of me with every step.

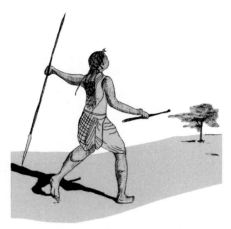

Aligned With The Earth

Movement is the coherent changing of shape. Energy is movement. If we are misaligned, movement of course is challenged. As you release the pelvis from the tight holdings of distorted musculature, muscle fibers are free to realign over bones and the legs can emerge longer into the earth. Pathways that have been energetically silenced awaken and the flow of energy along the conduits of the nervous system stream into new openings. Movement becomes a new journey.

Elders in walkers need the strength provided by the apparatus as the legs are not free to stream out of the pelvic floor and the spinal muscles are not free to elongate out of the pelvis. Hence the walker becomes the legs. I must say that I never saw an elder in Kenya, one who had lived truly with the earth, who was walking with the aid of a walker.

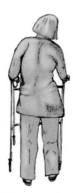

Shuffling on the Earth

Animals provide such a beautiful reminder of the movement patterns we hold deep in our cellular memory. When I watch the movement of horses, front and back legs streaming out of the pelvis, I feel a visceral connection to such a movement within me. Watching racehorses, it always appeared to me that the back legs were running backwards and the forward legs forward. I thought it to be an optical illusion and yet watching the Masai warriors running across the plains I saw and *felt* the same freedom of movement. The leg that was behind appeared to be climbing backwards out of the pelvis at the same time the front leg initiated the forward movement. How could I feel that same movement, both forward and backward at the same time?

"Walking is man's best medicine."
—Hippocrates

The same movement can be seen in big cats who fly across the African plains, movement unimpeded. Indeed, four-legged beings have a great advantage. The front legs actually have a job that our upper limbs no longer have. Becoming upright beings has the muscles of the upper torso challenged to stretch in ways we never needed to as a four legged. The innate knowledge that lives in our energetic system from our earlier ancestral forms is not readily accessed. Feeling the arms extend out of the pelvis in our upright walking movement has not been in our awareness. And yet, the upper torso plays a vital role in our postural carriage and movement through space.

Having witnessed and felt within myself my back leg walking backwards so that the psoas muscle is completely stretching the femur bone out of the pelvis, I can lift my torso up and out and allow the front leg to stream forward. The legs become a lot longer with all the space created between the bottom of the sacrum, the tailbone, thighs, and buttocks. The leg bones, free from entangled musculature, allow my feet to descend into the earth. I want to walk into the earth, not on it. How removed we have become from the home we live on, Earth, and the home we live in, our body.

While putting into movement (walking) what you have been learning in your unraveling stretches can be a challenge, you are holding the same instructions and map within your being. The clock is ever present. The pelvis and the legs must have space in between. The upper torso relies on this space to emerge up and out and hence space is created between each vertebra. The discs in between the vertebrae fill up that space and the muscles along the vertebral column do their job of stretching the spine. Remember, we want to

get taller as we age, not shorter. Weight-bearing while walking elongates the
spine. We stretch the free leg bones out of the pelvis, descending deeply into
the earth. Use your weight to move the earth beneath you.

With your back numbers flying open and relaxing the muscle fibers underneath the base of your buttocks, you have room to stretch the legs, using
so much more of your psoas and adductors along the inside of your thighs.
The psoas connection along the lumbar spine stretches your erector spinae
muscles. With the abdominals behind the pubic bone gently moving into
the low back, your sacral muscles elongate and space is created between the
sacrum and the lumbar, at the waist area.

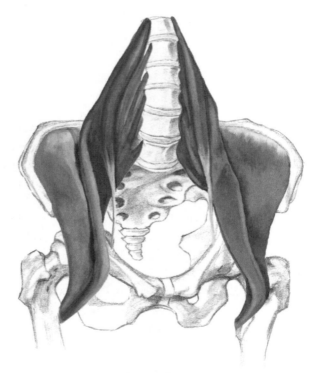

The Regal Psoas

To maintain the integrity of this structure in movement releases more
energy and creates possibility. We are opening up to receive so much more
information, allowing the light to inform us. We are free to see more, explore
more, be more of our intended design here in this lifetime. One of my stu-

dents remarked, upon lifting his upper body so smoothly out of his lower as his legs climbed so far out and down beneath the earth, "I feel so dignified." Walking with dignity—I like that.

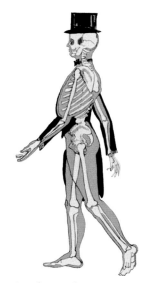

Walking Awake With Connection to Earth

WALKING AS IF YOU'VE NEVER WALKED BEFORE

Let's now walk as if you have never walked before, shaking up your neurology even more. As we incorporate everything we've just learned about the expansion of the pelvic floor into our well-known movement patterns, a whole lot of shakiness and confusion arises. The bones are now required to move you in new ways that are not yet incorporated into your energy body. You will feel off-balance, using new muscles, and that is a good indication that changes are happening for the better.

Practice walking not just inside, but outside, on softer earth or sand, and even barefoot when possible. Move that earth deeper underneath your feet. Your feet merge into the earth and your upper torso rises up out of the earth.

I want you to slow down this walking process, one step at a time. This slow-motion gait brings the awareness into the pelvis and the site of the perineum where we have been focusing so far.

When you first try this exercise, do so indoors, on a hard surface with bare feet.

A quick note on helpful props: You might want to walk near a wall or a railing so that your hand can have that support should you feel you need it. When I am practicing with a client I sometimes hold their hand and as we walk together they can feel more stability. You will be using parts of your musculature on your legs that have not stretched before, hence the wobbliness. You might want to invite a helpful friend in the beginning, to support you in feeling more of these places called into action.

Begin in your upright standing posture with everything you know now, creating the freedom in the base of the pelvis. 12 o'clock down, abdominals back, back numbers open, 6 o'clock down, sacrum elongating, "eyes behind the thighs" revealed, heels planted, lifting upper torso out of lower. By now, I have repeated this so many times I am hoping there is a little mantra going on in your body vocabulary! You are so firmly planted in the earth that taking one step forward should feel as if the leg initiating the movement has to lift the back foot way out of the earth as the front foot reaches way down into the earth.

> "Life is available only in the present. That is why we should walk in such a way that every step can bring us to the here and the now."
> —**Thich Nat Hanh**

Here you go. Bend your right knee and lift the foot off the floor slightly, an inch or two. If balance is immediately tricky, don't even lift the foot, just lighten the weight on the right side. Bring your right fingers to the very base of the buttocks, guiding the flesh open and back, so that the back right quadrant of the perineal clock, 6, 5, and 4 expands. Begin to walk the right leg forward, stretching it out of the open perineum. You will notice that as the leg that moves forward, to take a step, the fibers under the buttocks will want to join you in that movement, pulling under the buttocks. Use your right fingers to expand those fibers as you walk the leg forward, extending it down and out of the open pelvic floor.

Keep the abdominals in the back body, elongating your sacrum and lift your upper torso way up and out of the pelvic floor. The heel of the right foot reaches for the floor first and lands on the floor. The toes are still lifted. How far ahead you walk the right leg can and will vary as you want to feel more extension. For now, perhaps a foot will do.

Your left leg, the back leg, is still extending down and out behind you and now your left fingertips widen the flesh in the lower left quadrant of the clock, 6, 7, and 8. The fibers under your buttocks are now fanning back.

Watch the tendency for the "eyes under the thighs" to retreat under. They likely will!

Roll the toes of your right foot out of the arch of the foot, feeling the balls of the right toes land on the floor, and keep the base of your right buttock opening back. You can still have your fingers guiding those back right perineal numbers open. In fact, taking steps with this support is helpful as you will feel how the muscle fibers are dragged under your butt with your forward-moving leg bone.

The left leg is still in its upright standing posture and hasn't moved forward: in fact, opening those left perineal numbers provides the room for the leg to keep streaming out of the pelvic floor behind you.

Elongate your left (back) heel all the way down on the floor behind you.

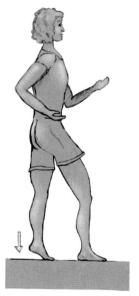

Walking Re-Minding Your Back Leg

The abdominals are in the back body, toward the sacrum, sliding those sacral muscles down toward the floor behind you. Remember that the extension of the sacral muscles gives you the space to lift your upper torso up and out. As in every other stretch, the space between the leg bones and the pelvic floor is what you want to expand.

Begin to take your weight forward onto the right foot, and the back left heel will begin to rise up. Before you think about walking your left foot and leg forward to take the next step, stretch the left heel back onto the floor again. Open those left back perineal numbers with your fingers if necessary. You have more room to stretch the inner left thigh musculature (your adductors and the psoas). The more you "weight bear," stretching the back leg down out of the pelvic floor into the earth behind you, the more you can lift, wiggle your upper torso out of the lower.

Now, as you lift the left heel (your back leg) and begin the movement of that leg forward, stretch the right leg out of the pelvis and the foot deeply into the floor. Use the floor. Move it below your foot as if moving it into the basement or the earth below. Reach *into* the earth.

Roll the abdominals up off the pelvic floor and feel the muscles along the spine elongate as your right leg reaches through the earth.

"A life is a moment in season. A life is one snowfall. A life is one autumn day. A life is the delicate, rapid edge of a closing door's shadow. A life is a brief movement of arms and of legs."
—Alan Lightman

Now you are ready to take the left leg forward out of your pelvis. Pressing the right leg into the earth, the left heel lifted, raise your left knee. Open those back left numbers and as you reach the leg out to the floor ahead, you will feel as if the floor is quite a long distance away from your foot. That is because the base of your buttocks and the back of the thigh muscles are still way back. This allows you to use those inner thigh muscles to elongate the left leg even more.

Now, reach the left heel onto the floor about a foot ahead of you. Your right leg is now the back leg. Keep stretching the right heel back and down behind you and open the back right numbers with fingers if necessary.

Roll the left toes forward out of the back of the left arch, as the bottom left perineal quadrant stays open. Bringing the ball of the toes onto the floor, begin to feel how the elongation of the toes connects all the way up into the upper inner thigh and ultimately into your pelvic floor. With the "belly in the back," elongate your upper torso out of the pelvic floor and stretch that left foot through the floorboards (or the earth, if practicing outside).

Before you begin to walk that right leg forward again, stretch open the back left quadrant of the perineal clock, 6, 7, and 8, those fibers emanating all the way out to the base of the buttocks. Don't let the "eye behind your thigh" on the left collapse under as you begin to walk forward. The back leg always needs a lot of attention as we tend to forget about it with the goal of walking forward.

Taking the weight onto your left (front) foot pressing through the floor, lift your right heel and then stretch the heel back down behind you again. You will feel the stretch along the quadriceps on that right leg and perhaps begin to feel the adductors and the psoas on that inner thigh as well.

When you lift the right heel again and begin your next step forward, remind those fibers under the right buttocks to fan open.

Take that step forward with your right leg, the heel placed out on the floor ahead of you. With 6, 5, 4 fanning open wide, the right leg has a long distance to reach the floor.

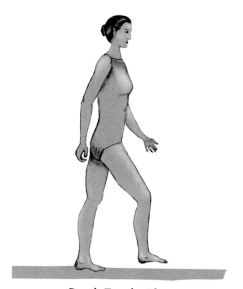

Reach For the Floor

Roll the right toes out of the back of the arch as if the toes were many inches away from the heel. The ball of the toes find the floor and the right foot begins to apply pressure into the floor. With the abdominals in the back body, the sacral muscles elongate back and down behind you.

Lift the head and the upper torso up out of the pelvis as the right leg begins to descend deeply into the earth (if you are walking outside), or through the floor (if inside.)

Slowing down your stride to this degree will have your balance quite confused and perhaps leave you rocky on the inside and outside of your feet. However, you will become aware of using muscles that you have not used before. Notice as you walk at this slow pace how each leg moves very differently out of your pelvic floor. My right droopy side has my right leg seemingly stuck up into my pelvis. I am consistently aware of the different actions that are necessary on each side to create a balanced walk.

Once you have practiced walking the legs out of the pelvis five times on each leg, bring the back leg forward alongside the front one and feel your stance, your balance, the amount of length you experience in your leg bones being supported through the floor into the earth. Notice if you feel a greater lift of your upper torso and the base of the buttocks. Readjust your standing posture to incorporate the new information your muscles have received. You can close your eyes (the ones in your head, not the ones behind the thighs!) for some breaths and notice what you experience.

WALKING UP A HILL AND UP
A FLIGHT OF STAIRS

Once you get used to walking on a flat plane, you might try walking up an incline, because moving that forward leg into the hill and lifting your upper torso up and out gives you more information. As the sacral muscles slide down the hill behind you, you are using the legs to climb you up the hill. Wearing a weighted backpack will make it more of a challenge to lift your upper torso out of the pelvis.

Your front leg moves the earth and you propel your upper torso out of the lower. Don't be in a rush to bring the back leg forward. Allow the front leg to do its job, keep those abdominals in the back and elongate your sacrum; then bring that back leg forward to do the same thing once again. Slow it way down.

Remember how in Chapter 2 I described the Sherpas in India and Nepal who carry their baskets weighing a hundred pounds, attached to a leather band across their foreheads, up the mountain trails? That weight does not pull them back down the mountain. They move their heads up and out of the pelvis, creating space for their upper torso to climb out of the lower. Once again, creating space in specific areas creates a greater, spaciousness throughout the entire energetic system, providing the freedom to move your structure with more elegance.

Imagine you are that Sherpa, moving your head into the leather band. That basket of weight is not sliding you back down the hill. Your sacral muscles are elongating down the mountain just like they do when you are in the squat while your upper torso is reaching up and out. Remember the image of the toddler in a squat. It's hard to imagine that you are in a squat going up the mountain but indeed you are. The child standing up from the squat sends the legs deep into the earth out of an open pelvis. The tail, the low back, is not curled under. There is room between the pelvis and the legs. Use that imaginary leather strap around your forehead and stretch the head out of the pelvic floor. You are now truly weight-bearing, the legs free to use the earth to stretch into.

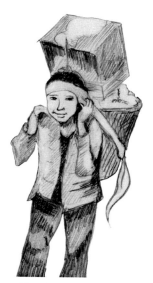

Climbing Up and Out

Practicing with stairs is most informative as well. Use the step you are taking, with open numbers, to move the stair deeply down under your foot.

It's almost like the feeling of being on an escalator, with the step retreating as you walk onto it. Envision lifting your upper torso way up and out as your leg slides out of your pelvis, just like the Sherpa with weight on his back. Your upper body is actually the weight you are lifting out of the pelvic floor.

PRACTICE EVERY DAY!

Walking is an activity we do every day, so you will have ample opportunities to practice bringing awareness to your movement. Notice how it is different with shoes and on different surfaces. Try taking the stairs rather than the elevator—it's a fabulous exercise for deepening your awareness of the importance of the legs to stretch the spine. Walk with elegance, remembering the Masai warriors. They walk *in* the earth. They walk with the earth. They are earth. We all have this capability as well.

For further resources to support your inquiry, including videos, guided audio exercise, and more visit:

www.corebodywisdom.com

CHAPTER 12

INFORMED MOVEMENT: RETHINKING SPORTS AND EXERCISE

"Dis-ease, joint and muscle pain, and limited movement range and vocabulary are all products of imbalance."

—Dr. Lulu Sweigard

IF YOU'VE BEEN practicing the postures and visualizations I've described in the last few chapters, I hope you are starting to feel a new awareness of your body, in particular the position of your pelvic floor. Now, I'd like to invite you to carry that awareness with you as you engage in movement. In the last chapter, we focused on an activity that almost all human beings practice, every day: walking. Now, we'll turn our attention to various forms of popular physical exercise and look at the problems these can cause and the possibility of approaching them in a new, informed way.

Because everybody is different, the way in which a particular sport affects you will be specific to your body's structure. In this chapter, I will introduce you to several of my clients, each of whom loves a particular form of exercise, and show you how I worked with them to bring their bodies into alignment and source their movement from the aligned pelvis.

In any sport you are playing, the position of the pelvic floor is vital to understand as you are moving. As you have experienced, just walking with an aligned pelvis is a major challenge. How much more challenging to stay in alignment as you run, jump, twist, lift, and swing!

We are an exercise-committed population; we might even say an exercise-addicted population. Indeed, a recent literature review concluded that while "exercise in appropriate quantity and of proper quality contributes to the preserve of our health," excessive exercise may be "harmful to our health."[62]

Our commitment to exercising despite a misaligned structure can create many challenges, as I discussed in Chapter 3. The world of chiropractic and physical therapy is booming, with clients who have injured themselves with fitness programs. Backs that have "gone out" (I love this terminology—as if our backs had a will of their own, and we played no part in the dysfunction), areas in the spine that may have been weakened way before a serious fitness practice evolved, are now in greater jeopardy of suffering even more intense ramifications. As discussed in Chapter 3, surgeries are plentiful, and studies show that hip replacements are rising among those in their thirties.

"To impose the posture on the body is wrong. The body has to find the posture using a finer energy."
—Dona Holleman, Yoga Practitioner

Misalignment in the pelvis causes havoc as we repetitively create any type of movement. Remember, movement is the coherent changing of shape. Movement created with an imbalanced structure creates changes in shape that are no longer coherent and aligned. Energy that is stuck in congested areas prevents movement with ease. When one area of the body experiences discomfort due to the effects of misaligned muscles the entire energy system is put on alert. Other areas begin to compensate for those that can no longer perform like they once did, yet the desire to keep running, golfing, playing tennis, or biking is strong, and other muscles have to be called in to take over for the weakened ones. So driven are we by our cultural ideals of physical perfection that we press on, regardless. This diverted energy creates havoc for the entire structural field.

Many of my clients are very dedicated to their health and fitness—so much so that they are inclined to continue to exercise regardless of physical injury. In many instances, when they show up seeking help and care in my practice, they have some recognition of when an injury occurred that led to the snowball effect. Yet they made the choice to push through and adjust to the current physical story because the thought of stopping was terrifying to them. Unraveling the distortions that led to the original injury, and even before that, to the original movement patterns, can open a Pandora's box of feelings, unraveling deep emotions held within the muscle-fiber cells.

Stories held in the cellular history of the physical structure all rise up. Unraveling the distortion in the musculature awakens much more than the recent injury.

Injuries are teachers, shadows and confusions unraveling, energy releasing as if from a river dammed up in protection. There is a surge of energy that wants to be expressed, new currents penetrating through the tension of the old patterns. There is a chaotic reorganization of the cell structure as the old congested alignment is threatened. As the new patterns are introduced, muscles and bones are confused and the structure exists in an in-between state of alignment—not in the old and not in the new. Very confusing.

Our more extreme sports tend to be reserved for the young and limber, and they can mask their symptoms for many years and still make a comeback many times after injuries. However, those of you that have been athletes know that your old injuries seem to rear up many years later, and with many new layers of distortion apparent as the torqued, twisted muscle has kept wrapping around the bones over time. Baseball and football players certainly have this experience, as do gymnasts.

"JUST GET ME BACK ON THE GOLF COURSE!"

My client Dennis is a successful businessman who lives for golf. When he was recommended to my practice, we spoke on the phone and I asked him what he wanted to achieve through our work. "Just get me back on the golf course!" he said emphatically.

He had not even considered how his physical story had evolved to the point where he could no longer walk eighteen holes; he actually couldn't even walk nine. Why his swing put him in excruciating pain wasn't even on the list of things he wanted to know. Like most people, he wasn't that interested (prior to our meeting) in exploring how he had come to this painful place he now lived in; he just wanted the problem to go away. "Let's fix it," he said.

Happily, for me, Dennis has a great sense of humor. He also has a high tolerance for pain and for years, even as his body spoke to him through its increasing discomfort, he simply kept going. As long as he was able to compete, and to develop satisfying relationships on the course, he made it work—until it didn't.

When I met Dennis, his posture was seriously challenged and he was barely able to even walk on one leg. The droop to one side was so prominent that his knees had been ailing him for years. He would go from one medical specialist to the next as his herniated disc became ever more herniated. Surgery was definitely an option if it meant he could get back on the golf course. He had tried surgery before but his old movement patterns that kept exacerbating his misalignment began to create further distortion and pain.

We talked about the beginnings of a body story such as his, which is, of course, not uncommon. As a young athlete he pushed his body relentlessly. High on the results of winning in competitive sports, he never considered attending to the resulting pain. Being in pain seemed an inevitable byproduct for him, as for all of his friends. As he traced his body story, he realized how his pain had evolved over time. He had always been involved in sports and his posture was always a challenge, he said. Like most of us living in our structures over many years (Dennis is in his sixties), we tend not to question what feels uncomfortable. It is just what is, and it is familiar. Doctors told Dennis that "at his age" these things are to be expected.

"Tell me, what is it you plan to do with your one wild and precious life?"

—Mary Oliver

Dennis worked hard at coming to new understanding and doing the practices I suggested. He realized how dramatically he tucked the muscle fibers under his buttocks causing the thigh bones to retreat from the back to the front, which in turn pulled his pelvis forward, and caused the other side to respond with a major twist. He was able to sense the source of his pain for himself. The initial injury wasn't in his back, the way he'd always thought.

When did he start to not be able to grow the legs out of his pelvis? He had no idea that they weren't. As we worked, he became very aware that he could not stretch his legs out of his pelvis and stand upright with a pelvis so intensely tucked under. This scenario for so many years, ever since his boyhood, created his herniated disc, which became ever more herniated. His upper body was literally collapsing onto the disc. Putting an intense twist onto that story became the nightmare he was now experiencing the result of.

As we continued our work together, Dennis began to open up the floor of his pelvis and understand how the fibers retreating were further exacerbating the disturbance in the pelvis, his legs, and the muscles of the back. He learned through practice how to keep these areas expanded. His main fear when looking ahead to getting back on the green was, "What if I lose the power in my swing?"

I explained to him that in the realignment of muscle over bone, muscles that had been hiding behind the layers of distortion and never used would now be called into action, with the possibility of creating even more strength. It takes courage to undo an old dysfunctional, painful pattern, and trust that what is coming can be even better.

Dennis and I broke down the movements as he practiced the basic stretches that gave him freedom in the pelvic floor. Through specific stretches that mimicked the twists in golf, he began to connect with the feeling that the golf club was an extension of his arm, evolving out of the pelvic floor. He learned that the twist required to get the power to have that ball fly far and on target was generated from a much deeper place in his body. The more his pelvis opened, the more expanded his sacral area became, and the more space between the bottom of the sacrum and the upper thighs, the stronger his swing.

All movement emerges out of the pelvis, as do all twists. I am always amazed to watch golfers and the differences in their swing depending on their alignment. I have watched golfers who have the hips perfectly aligned as they take that club across their body and it is truly beautiful to watch. But I have also watched golfers like Dennis, and it is a painful sight.

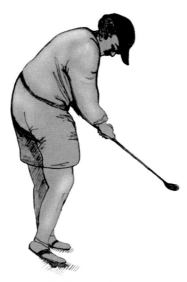

Golfing with Pain

When Dennis began to create the space in the pelvic floor, he could feel the power in his legs and automatically felt his upper body climb higher up. "I am taller," he remarked. The realignment of Dennis' structure did not happen in just a few sessions, as the musculature needed time to adjust to new possibilities. However, his awareness was sparked immediately in the very first session. Through his practice in our sessions and on his own, within three to four months his realignment was starting to take hold and inform his neurology. Now his body was finding a new attunement and he noticed that when he moved without awareness of his old patterns pain would arise. Dennis did not have to give up golf, he had to give up living in his old distorted patterns.

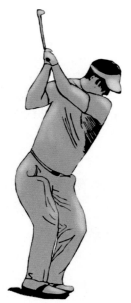

At One with the Club

If you, like Dennis, love golf but experience pain on the course, the most important exercise you can do is to become intimate with your standing position (see Chapter 7), because all the information you need about your muscular dysfunction is present in your stance. Once you put dramatic twists on top of your misaligned structure, it is inevitable that you will experience pain. Learning to stand on two feet needs to be your first priority.

A SERIOUS CYCLIST

When Phil first came to see, me his lament was that because of the pain in his hip and leg, he was unable to bike the many miles in practice and competition that he had built up to over the years. His "extreme" biking regime had included biking across the United States. He was very fit, strong, and motivated. I would not say that Phil was addicted to his sport; his sport did not define who he is. He is an athlete and a most balanced being, but he loves his sport and was anxious to regain his strength so that he could cycle long-distance again.

He had no idea how his pain had come about. Within a very short time it had become so intense that he could only bike for short distances, if at all. At our first meeting, I could see immediately that he was not standing on two legs, and the pelvic floor muscles, the quadriceps muscles, and the sacral musculature were all pulling him over to one side. The twist—the scoliosis—in his lower spine was apparent.

After a few sessions awakening the muscle-fiber cells to a new pattern, Phil realized where the deeply raveled fibers in and around the perineum were pulling him out of alignment. The repetitive movement of the legs turning those bike pedals, with the collapse of his pelvis on one side, were reinforcing this distortion. This realization had light bulbs going off for him. However, the real breakthrough came when we started working together in his home studio, where he could actually show me how he sits in the bike saddle, how he rides. He placed his bike on a standing platform so that he could simulate riding out in the world. It was fascinating for me to actually witness him leaning over to one side of the seat and see how the opposite leg was being pulled up into his pelvic floor. That leg could not stretch deep into the pedal and the leg that was doing all the work had to deal with the opposite side of the body leaning over to that already overworked side.

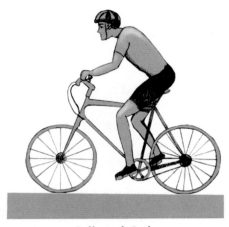

Collapsed Cyclist

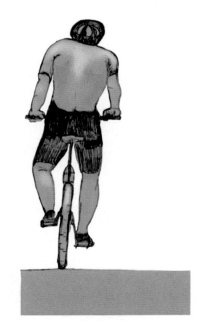

Perineum Unbalanced In the Saddle

The journey he embarked on was learning to lift out of that collapsed side as he unraveled the confused, twisted muscle fibers in the perineum, all the way out into the pelvic bowl, and farther out into the musculature on his thighs. The tucked under position of his buttocks with the perineal clock numbers retreating under had his lower back in great jeopardy as he reached for the handlebars. There was no way that the spine could stretch out of the pelvic floor, for the misaligned pelvis prevented the psoas from performing at its optimum. The sinking of the spine down into the pelvis put another extreme tension on his lower body.

As I supported Phil to awaken places of disturbance, he began to shift weight from deep in the pelvis so that his "hiked up" leg began to have the freedom to elongate out and reach way down into the earth. He could reach into that pedal and follow the motion all the way around. What a relief for the droopy side. As he realigned and awakened the adductors and the psoas, his spinal muscles began to unravel as well. He could climb his spine out of the pelvis and release the center of the perineum down into the center of the seat. Now, when he rides, he is doing a squat on the bike seat!

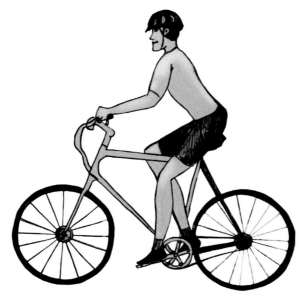

A Balanced Perineum In The Saddle

For anyone who likes to cycle, it is important to recognize which side of your pelvic floor has more weight on the seat. Over time, the musculature on the opposite side on the leg and along the spine has nowhere to go but towards the side that is dropping. Practicing the standing posture and learning your specific misalignment will transfer to your bicycle seat.

Phil rarely has pain anymore as he bikes. When he forgets and defaults to his imbalance and habitual movement patterns, he now has a map and a protocol to bring him to his next unraveling. I continue to work with Phil occasionally, whenever I visit his home city. Each time I work with his structure, I marvel at the new spaces that he has created with his devotion to his practice. He becomes so much more embodied as his energy being has more space to be at home. He is also an avid backpacker and the same scenarios play out in his structure when he is not attentive to his "droopy" side in his hiking. With a heavy backpack collapsing him into his low back, he has learned to open the areas around his perineum, his upper torso having the freedom to lift him up and out of the collapse. He recognizes that the side of the body he defaults to prevents him from using that opposite leg to climb up a mountain. He now knows he will be able to keep hiking and biking for a long time.

What Phil understands is that as the muscle fibers begin to let go, as space is created and his energy body expands, there is always more unraveling to come. There are always more awakenings, more freedom, and more connections to be made far beyond the physical plane. This home we live in is a never-ending field of information that is teaching us the depth of who we are. With more freedom comes more awareness.

"JUST KEEP RUNNING, GINNY!"

"Just keep running, Ginny." It was the eighties, and these sarcastic words came from my first serious yoga teacher, Larry Hatlett in Palo Alto, California. I had been complaining to him after class about my knees, and he told me in no uncertain terms how to ensure that they would just keep getting worse. As he knew, in those days, I was very wedded to my running practice, had even trained to run some marathons. It just felt good—until it didn't. I didn't notice the tension when I was running, but I always felt it in Larry's advanced yoga class. Certain poses made it perfectly clear that pain in various places was becoming a normal Wednesday evening lament.

Yoga opened the doors to what I was not seeing and clearly feeling. However, back in those days I had not yet discovered the source of all of my misalignment and I was overriding it to get into the postures.

I now appreciate what my wise teacher was trying to tell me. Running puts our out-of-whack-structure into a most tenuous situation. You have only to watch runners out there on the streets to see the variety of postural patterns. When you see an aligned body glide across the earth, it is energetically satisfying to witness. But when you see a twisted, distorted, imbalanced body shuffling or pounding along, it's painful just to watch.

Personally, I had no idea that my entire right upper torso was drooping into my right leg and that foot was striking heavier into the ground. I never made the connection with the fact that I had sprained the same ankle badly three times over the years.

As yoga and my deep transformative study became ever more important, I stopped running and was able to research my imbalances with greater awareness. Slowing way down, I noticed my inability to get into certain postures without pain. My standing pose, tadasana, began to inform me as to the misalignment of the musculature around my bones. As I unraveled, my old injuries began to inform me. I was feeling the old chapters in my body story come alive. Now I could understand how weakness around my ankles created my three sprained ankles from a teenager onward.

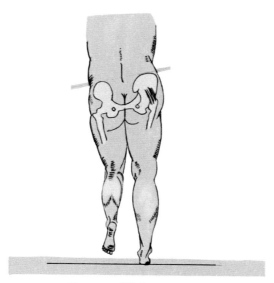

Running With Distortion

Walking and hiking became a much more enjoyable stretch, and for a while extreme hiking at great altitude was most exciting. This activity became a study of alignment, as the demands on my body awakened me to what was required, moment by moment. My initial patterns, ingrained within, were never far in the background. The past does indeed inform the present and allow the future to present new ways of being. I can include the past as it continues to inform me as to my misalignment and transcend the past with my new tools of transformation.

Over the years, I have worked with many runners, and my own experience informs me as I help them. When Peter came to my Pelvic Floor Awakening Yoga class, he immediately informed me that he had recently had a knee replacement. An avid runner, he wanted to get back to running in the very best way he could. He had been to physical therapy as per the prescription after surgery and had heard that my classes dealt with understanding the original story within the structure—the source of what may have made his knee vulnerable to begin with.

It did not take more than a few moments to see how Peter was collapsing and that his tucked-under tail and the extreme movement forward of his femur bones prevented him from straightening his legs at all. Of course, like most of us Westerners, he was profoundly leaning into one side. That poor knee did not have a chance, as he never used the musculature on the inner knee to stretch the lower leg into the earth. Most of us cannot feel the lower leg bones stretch out from an open space in the knee area because the forward movement of the pelvis creates the inability to use the leg muscles.

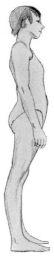

Hyperextension

In just months, Peter was learning about his perineal clock and practicing stretches to open and awaken the areas that were hiding in shadow, preventing him from extending his legs and his upper body out of the pelvis. He began to recognize how the distortion in the floor of his pelvis had created his collapse and the fall of his upper torso on to one side of his body. The muscles around the challenged kneecap did not have the ability to perform as the muscles of the inner thigh were not activated. Understanding this dysfunctional pattern, with new stretches to inform him, he could feel the tension created around his knee and learned to awaken those inner thigh muscles.

I see Peter often when I return to his home city. His posture continues to transform as his musculature realigns as a result of his committed practice. He loves to run and now knows how to keep his body aligned so he can keep running for a very long time.

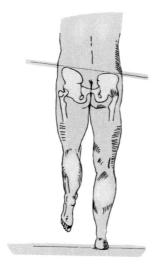

Running With Ease

If you are a runner, it's critical that you don't "just keep running" without awareness of your own distortion. Running with misalignment, pounding into the earth with the distortions in the pelvic floor, puts an incredible stress on the entire structure. Awareness of how your body walks on the earth is vital to understanding what happens when you then engage your structure in a faster pace.

Most serious runners stretch their legs and sometimes their spines before and after. However, they may have no idea that they are falling into one side of their body. As long as the pattern does not create very much pain, they keep going.

Again, I suggest practicing the standing posture to find out how your body's challenges are affecting your running, so that when you begin to run, you are aware of which leg takes most of the weight. Elongating the sacral muscles while in movement takes focus, the legs streaming out of the pelvis with the upper torso rising up is a challenge. Gravity has you collapsing into your lower torso, into your low-back.

As you become more attuned to your old patterns, practicing the other stretches I've shared will help you become further enlightened as to where sticky places (muscles literally stuck on the bones) prevent openings. You can then begin to integrate your new awareness into your running.

YOGA

In my very intense and thorough training as an Iyengar Yoga teacher, I took very seriously the instruction from B.K.S. Iyengar that "seeing and understanding bodies" is of the utmost importance. Over the years, as I recognized my inability to perform poses on my right side with the same freedom as on my left I began to question, on a much deeper level, where my imbalance was actually arising from. I had to see and understand my own structural stories and how pain manifested before I could actually see another's.

What I noticed as I watched people practicing postures was the lack of connection about where in the body each asana originates. Most people attempt to *im*pose the pose on their distorted bodies. Actually these poses already live within us, and true yoga involves removing the distortion to discover the pose from within. I am reminded of Michelangelo's famous unfinished sculptures, the Prisoners or the Slaves. They line the hallway leading to the perfectly finished specimen of his David. When I visited the Galleria dell'Accademia in Florence, Italy, I was completely taken with these bodies encased within the stone that seemed to be emerging and yet could not get out. I experienced a visceral recognition within myself that I had been in the same dilemma, emotionally and physically.

In my experience practicing yoga, I felt I needed to find that place from where the pose originated, and yet I could tell I had no access to specific places deep within my pelvic floor. I was stuck inside and most often could not feel the birth of the pose from deep within. I was indeed my own prisoner within my structure. Creating those spaces all around the perineal circle, out into the perineum and entire pelvic floor, gifted me the emergence of movement from this deep awakening place in my base.

In yoga, that which is manifest within can emerge with grace. Rather than "wearing" a posture on your structure, see if you can discover how your fingers stretch out of a completely open perineum to unravel the arm that is of course connected to the spine and how the spine emerges, the head crawling out and the legs as well.

A yoga practice is the perfect place to learn how your own body is constructed. As you stretch into triangle pose, for example, feel how the back leg cannot fully extend out of the pelvis, because the back numbers around the perineum are tucked under and the "eyes behind the thighs" cannot peek out. You are literally in a vice in poses if the pelvis is not free and the legs are not separated from the muscles, tying you up in knots.

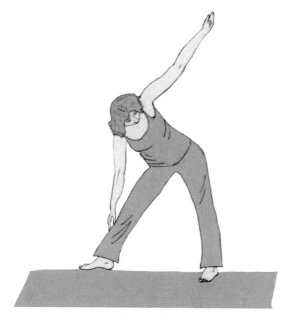

Yoga with Pain

For most people, the tuck of the pelvis is so dramatic that in yoga postures, as in any movement, you are going to come up against the inability to stretch your legs out of the pelvic floor. The stretches you've learned in this book will inform every yoga pose you practice, including backbends, which indeed present a great challenge. To stand on our feet with our legs elongating out of the pelvis is the constant practice. Knowing how to create more space will take you deeper into a more satisfying practice.

Creating a backbend from the floor of the pelvis, while having the back body surrender into an imaginary hammock is truly an exercise in letting go of control. If you have experienced bridge pose (the precursor to the full "wheel" backbend, where the shoulders and arms remain on the floor while the pelvis lifts up), you know how difficult it is to keep the buttock muscles soft and allow the front of the perineum to drop, deepening the spaces at the very top of the thighs, the root, where the femur and the pelvis meet. There is such a tendency to squeeze the buttock muscles together and thrust the pelvis up as the sacrum comes off the floor. Making space this way, hanging the sacral muscles into the imaginary fabric of the hammock, allows room for the leg bones to emerge and the feet move into the earth. Even in a backbend you are standing on your feet in the earth, through the earth.

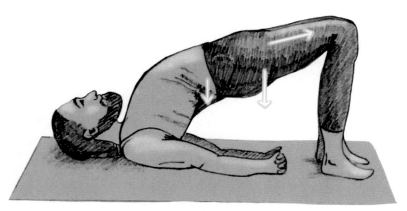

Bridge with Surrender

The ribcage breathes downward away from the upper chest and the lumbar spine receives the fullness of the breath. You are hanging completely into the back body, as if you are surrendering into the hammock fabric. The spine then wiggles out of the pelvis elongating and the chest lifts beautifully because it can. The neck elongates and the head is free to emerge as well.

Remember how I explained in Chapter 7 that your standing pose, in correct alignment, is in fact a backbend. The release into the back body in your standing posture (called mountain pose, or *tadasana*, in yoga), is the same movement as the full bend. As the sacrum releases into the hammock of your back body, all the musculature surrenders off the bones and the leg bones have permission to release away from the tight holding of the quadriceps.

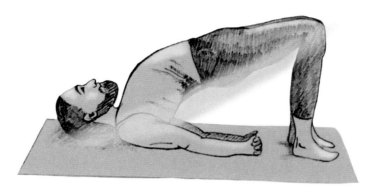

Deeper Letting Go

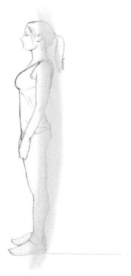

Always In the Hammock

The abdominals behind the pubic bone are received into the sacrum. As the ribcage breathes downward and the abdominals behind the pubic bone move gently into the back body, the sacrum is given permission to slide off.

This moment may seem like a conundrum, as we are so tempted to forcefully lift the chest, tightening the gluteus muscles and causing the ribcage to fly up into a military posture stance. Play with this and watch as the back numbers tighten under the butt and the anus constricts. With an open perineal area, the legs emanate from the pelvic floor and the spinal muscles wave all the way up and out. So much space is created that like a hand lifting from the bottom of the pelvic floor all the way up to the sternum and upper chest, the chest is lifted right up off the inner structure. When the ribcage breathes downward, the sacral muscles elongate and drop as if releasing into a squat, and the legs elongate even more, moving deep below the earth.

This is indeed a backbend that could now continue to move into a full wheel, eventually from standing, for the legs are rooting ever deeper into the earth. You may not personally feel inclined to try that rather extreme pose, and certainly it's not advisable for a beginner without guidance, but it is a good visualization for experiencing how elongating the spinal muscles creates spaces between each and every vertebra.

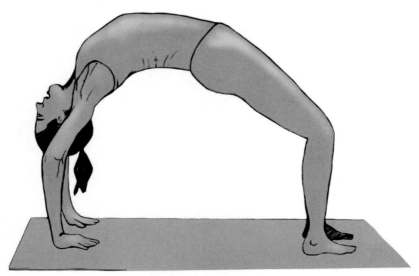

Surrender Even More

OTHER SPORTS

Tennis. Weight training. Baseball. Football. Swimming. Rowing. Archery. The list goes on. Each of these beloved sports and many others—from the most popular to the most obscure—can be challenging for a body that is out of alignment.

I have had the honor and privilege of teaching an Olympian to be, Katharine, for a short time. She was in the process of becoming the world-class rower she now is. When she first came to see me as a high school student, she was leaning over to one side of her body. Like twisting in golf, rowing encourages one side of the body to develop much differently than the other.

As Katharine showed me her positioning, I quickly realized that she was collapsing into one side of her buttocks on the bench in the boat, the side on which she rowed. Hence she could not achieve the full strength and length of her arms out of the floor of the pelvis. The opposite leg was not rooted through the floor of the boat providing the "ballast" needed for every powerful stroke. Once Katharine could feel her base she was quick to plant herself on both "eyes behind the thighs" and feel the new depth at the root of the formerly elevated femur bone. In tune with her energy, she was able to then incorporate the pelvic floor position in all of her training sessions; running, weight lifting, and more. Watching her at the Rio Olympics, deep in her craft, in her artistry, was a true honor.

Whenever I watch sports, I am observing bodies that are highly developed but often highly distorted as well. For example, while watching baseball, I marvel at the length of an arm, elongated so far out of the shoulder girdle to propel that ball. I have actually "felt" the possibility of such length in my own body. I've also noticed how the distortion in the pelvic floor prevents optimal freedom in the upper torso as the players twist to swing the bat and leap to strike out a runner.

Taking my granddaughter to swim club, I would walk through the local tennis club, and wince while watching so many older men and women demanding that their bodies perform. After years of living in distorted patterns, they are trying to create movement from their old body memories, when they had more freedom to run and jump. But it's not only the older ones among us. Speaking of my granddaughter, I watch her and her friends riding horses, and notice how the weight falls to one side of the saddle. I'm sure this imbalance is not doing them, or the horses, any favors!

To perform any movement with grace and attunement, knowing your body's patterns as you move is vital, and is an investment in your physical future. To awaken to the places in our structure that have been hiding out is the beginning of yet another opportunity to be present in body, emotion, and intellect. The "attuned" body has access to more energy and creates more space in which to experience the joy of movement

For further resources to support your inquiry, including videos, guided audio exercise, and more visit:

www.corebodywisdom.com

CHAPTER 13

ALIGNING WITH YOUR DESTINY

"We are star dust . . . and we are all one, in that sense."
—Edgar Mitchell

ALIGNMENT. IT IS a word with many layers of meaning. What does it truly mean to be aligned, physically, emotionally, mentally, and spiritually? What does it mean to be *in tune* with life?

As we've seen in these pages, the physical cannot be separated from the emotional, mental, and the spiritual. Where there is distortion in the body, there is also energetic misalignment that manifests at many levels. Ultimately, I believe each of us is here to align with our destiny—to make a unique contribution to the evolutionary process that only we can make. It can manifest as your unique professional calling, a craft or artistic expression, a spiritual journey, or your presence in service to others—children, a partner, society, or the planet. I think of this destiny as a contract that we accepted as part of the conditions of our arrival in this physical form. What it means to fulfill that contract will look different for every person, but what I have observed, over and over again, is that the freedom of the physical form is critical to our ability to do whatever it is we are here to do.

I've already shared several examples of this. Judith, the artist whose story I shared in Chapter 1, experienced depression and the loss of her creativity as she became imprisoned within her twisted body, and was able to release that creative energy onto the canvas again as she unraveled her physical structure. Each of the athletes I introduced in the previous chapter found a new level of mastery in their chosen sport as they created more space to move out of the pelvis.

I have worked with many other people who clearly have life work that depends on their physicality. I have had the honor to experience their "art" and how they have manifested more of their creativity—their unique genius—through dropping deeply into the pelvic floor and becoming present in their base.

Sophia is a viola virtuoso with one of the most renowned orchestras in America. She came to me because she needed to explore her sitting posture and how that affected her playing. Orchestra members sit for most of their day, in the hall, or at home practicing. When I attend a concert, as I enjoy the music, I always look at the posture of the musicians on stage and know how much pain they must be feeling in their spine with the collapse of their upper torso into the pelvic floor.

> "The point of power is always in the present moment."
> —Louise Hay

Most are not using their legs while sitting to elongate the spine out of the pelvis. (Remember how, in the sitting pose in Chapter 7, I explained that we still need to use the legs for weight bearing even when we are seated?) Sophia brought her viola to my studio. As she played and I adjusted her pelvis so that she was seated forward on the front of her perineum with the back of the perineum descending, the sound lifted up out of her pelvis filling the entire room, all the way up to my thirty-foot ceilings. Sophia had for many of her adult years sought out modalities to support her body to be strong and flexible in her journey to the level of expertise she now embodies. She knew there was more space to be had, more sound to birth forth.

A similar client was Roland, a jazz musician. As a horn player, he is standing most of the time. He also is an avid yoga practitioner and now teacher. He realized that the misalignment in the pelvic floor had him clearly standing on only one leg and with his pelvis thrust forward. Listening to his sound birthing from a new depth of space as I moved him gently into anatomical position, my heart was taken on a journey with him.

You may be thinking what I'm saying applies just to athletes and overtly creative people. In fact, it has been my observation that many professions and activities depend on this awareness as to where the pelvis is placed in relation to the legs and the spine. Massage therapists, for example, are literally using their own structure to awaken their clients'. Many have come to me, along with physical therapists, in search of understanding as to why their bodies are in such pain. It is not only the athletes who have misused and misaligned structures.

In the last years, I have worked with two dentists who have told me about the extreme pain they are in most every moment they are working. Leaning over the client, as well as twisting to one side has their musculature deranged. So many years of twisting the fibers around the bones, causing the bones to swivel with the ever-moving muscle fibers, has caused havoc. Both of these professionals have come to work with me and have achieved an understanding of how each of their situations has progressed to the current state.

Whatever form its expression takes, alignment of body and soul is the path of awakening I am speaking of. Being in tune, like an instrument, so that the sound of the universe can speak through your human form is the ultimate goal of this work. You may not even know the potential that is trapped within your own being, waiting to be released, until you begin the work of alignment.

It may seem grandiose to imagine that through healing distortion in the physical structure the doors and windows of perception can widen to possibility and creativity you had no idea was there. But when you remember that the root of the distortion, the perineum, is also the source of our beginning, the place where the light of consciousness arrived in this physical home, it makes sense that unraveling this place unleashes tremendous spiritual power.

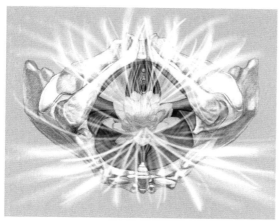

Awakening Consciousness

It is my belief that we each chose to be here, to go through the entanglements, through the layers of story, through the embryological stages of development, to be informed, to allow a greater consciousness to teach us and join
this magnificent energetic river of divine truth.

How does healing the stories, the karmic conditioning inherited from
thousands and thousands of years that lives in every cell of your being provide
the opportunity for the light of your soul to *in*form you, *re*form you, *re*mind
you of who you are? Culture lives in the depth of your tissues, leading you
to make decisions based on beliefs that you have inherited. To take all the
constraints off, undo the belief systems that have formed your physicality, and
experience your divine essence is a passionate life journey.

The pelvic floor is also the home of nurturing, of safety and security. The
deepest feminine principle resides here. How can we be in tune, in alignment
with the original flow when we have never felt safe, and perhaps never even
knew what safety meant? When stress, the weight of carrying pain, be it physical and or emotional, is liberated from the cell structure and we land softly
in the base, the pelvic floor, we can come home to a deeper safety. From here,
we can begin to partner with our energetic core that has been lying dormant
for so long, waiting for us to peek through the shadows and heal our ancient
and current lifetime challenges.

I must remind you, once again, that this journey of embodiment is not
an easy one. Opening places that have been held so tightly closed can feel
scary. Opening to those places in the musculature where you might believe
the pain lies, only to find that the chords of entanglement lie elsewhere and
that those chords have been architecturally designed by you, can bring forth
feelings that are perhaps quite uncomfortable. An awareness that has been
lying dormant is now finding the space to feel. That is why I always say that
this journey takes commitment. Awakening is not for the faint of heart. To
become coherent and congruent in a being that is fraught with fear of being
fully embodied is not possible.

Despite the challenges, I hope that everything you've learned and experienced as you've journeyed through these pages with me has given you the
inspiration and courage to keep going—not just for your own sake but for
a higher purpose. Aligning with your destiny has clear implications for not
only you personally, but for humanity as a whole. We live in a society that

is ever-more connected by technology, and all of our spiritual and religious teachings tell us that we are all connected at the deepest level of our consciousness as well. We are no longer able to live in the small bubbles we have been accustomed to retreating to. We are a global community made up of all of us living in confusion and distortion, perceptions skewed, beliefs guiding us and misguiding us.

How can physical alignment, coming home to center, to our base of safety, unleashing our passion and creativity, serve humanity? Recognizing higher purpose, living in a structure that is becoming whole through the journey of belonging to something far greater, cannot help but produce greater awareness. Energy unleashed from the source of divine movement can only have divine consequences for our global population. As the fear within the cell structures is released, as *attunement* realigns and reorders us, we become ever greater expressions of divine truth, able and ready to join this next evolutionary wave of transformation.

For those of us who are fortunate enough to have the freedom, the resources, and the time to devote to our own healing, I see no good reason for not achieving the magnificence we truly are. I see this time we are living in one in which the gates are wide open in ways they have never been before. Not all will choose to walk through now, and not all will have the support necessary to do so. However, many more beings are creating relational fields that support personal and global healing with heightened responsibility.

Awakening to one's destined life is available to everyone no matter the circumstances one is born into. Our shadows are here to inform us, guide us, and ultimately free us. The layers we have constructed to keep ourselves hidden and protected peel away, and we catch glimpses of the magnificence we truly are. This journey that we take together in safety and trust creates the relational fields that support personal and global healing with heightened responsibility.

My wish for you, as you continue on this journey to physical freedom is to begin to experience the many layers of possibility that have been lying dormant within your cell structure. On the journey back home, the journey to belong, to be embraced and to take precious care, you will meet yourself in new ways, with renewed life force—connected, coherent, and congruent in body, emotions, mind, and spirit.

PRAYER

In the silence of my heart I Am
In the silence I hear thy name
From the pool of silence in my heart I hear thy whisper
In the beauty of the world I see thy face
I am grateful for what I see and for what is revealed to me
I am grateful for what stays hidden
For this is thy will and therefore I am here now and forever
Amen

—Thomas Hübl

ABOUT THE ILLUSTRATORS

PATRICIA MALCOLM CREATED all of the medical illustrations in this book, as well as many of the other images. You can learn more about her work at www.PatMalcolm.com and contact her at earth7artist@gmail.com.

Additional images were created by Susan Viets, stviets@gmail.com.

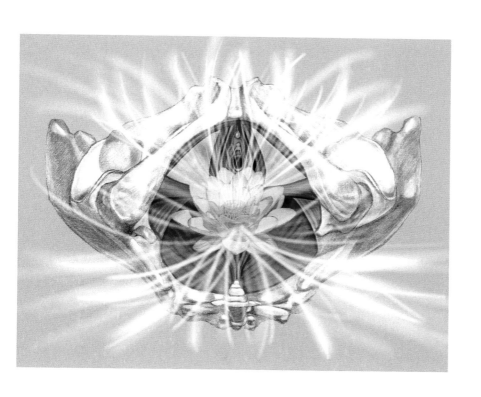

ENDNOTES

1. Thomas Hübl, Timeless Wisdom Training session, 2016
2. Andrew Harvey, *The Hope: A Guide to Sacred Activism* (Hay House, Inc. 2009), 39-42.
3. Thomas Hübl, Timeless Wisdom Training session, 2016
4. David Wise, Ph.D &Rodney Anderson, M.D., *A Headache in the Pelvis: A New Understanding and Treatment for Prostatitis and Chronic Pelvic Pain Syndrome* (National Center For pelvic Pain Research, 2012), 106.
5. Ibid, 126.
6. Ibid, 125.
7. Philip Beach, *Muscles and Meridians, The Manipulation of Shape* (Churchill Livingston Elsevier, 2010), 3.
8. Ibid, 187.
9. Ibid, 28.
10. Ibid, 36.
11. Ibid, 37.
12. Ibid, 37.
13. Ibid, xi.
14. Phillip Beach, "The Contractile Field-A Model of Human Movement, Part 1," *Journal of Bodywork and Movement Therapies*, Volume 11, Number 4, 308-17, October 2007
    http://www.bodyworkmovementtherapies.com/article/S1360-8592(06)00118-5/abstract
15. Phillip Beach, http://www.phillipbeach.com/contractile_fields.html)
16. Phillip Beach, *Muscles and Meridians, The Manipulation of Shape* (Churchill Livingston Elsevier, 2010), 39.
17. "2016 Yoga in America, Study Conducted by *Yoga Journal* and Yoga Alliance Reveals Growth and Benefits of the Practice," Yoga Alliance, https://www.

yogaalliance.org/Home/Media_Inquiries/2016_Yoga_in_America_Study_Conducted_by_Yoga_Journal_and_Yoga_Alliance_Reveals_Growth_and_Benefits_of_the_Practice

18. Dr. Raza Awan, "Yoga Can Lead to Hip Injuries," CBC News/Health, November 15, 2013, http://www.cbc.ca/news/health/yoga-can-lead-to-hip-injuries-1.2427134

19. William J. Broad, "Women's Flexibility is a Liability (in Yoga)," *The New York Times Sunday Review/News Analysis*, November 2, 2013
http://www.nytimes.com/2013/11/03/sunday-review/womens-flexibility-is-a-liability-in-yoga.html

20. American Academy of Orthopaedic Surgeons, March 14, 2014 http://newsroom.aaos.org/media-resources/Press-releases/25-million-americans-living-with-an-artificial-hip-47-million-with-an-artificial-knee.htm

21. Dr. Mark Pagnano, "Number of Hip Replacements Has Skyrocketed: Report," WebMD, February 12, 2015, http://www.webmd.com/arthritis/news/20150212/number-of-hip-replacements-has-skyrocketed-us-report-shows#1

22. Young Adult Hip Service, Barnes Jewish Hospital, http://www.barnesjewish.org/Medical-Services/Orthopedic-Care/Joint-Preservation-Resurfacing-and-Replacement-Hip-and-Knee/Young-Adult-Hip-Service

23. Robert Weisman, "Can surgery help you stay in the game? Demand for hip and knee replacement rises," *Boston Globe*, February 26, 2012 https://www.bostonglobe.com/business/2012/02/26/demand-for-knee-and-hip-replacement-growing-among-class-young-actives/Vu7EE0lUhBvDJNcHaKJBRP/story.html

24. Harrison Fryette, D.O., *Principles of Osteopathic Technic.* (Academy of Applied Osteopathy, First Edition, 1954)

25. Richard S. Bercik, M.D. Yale School of Medicine, *Female Urinary Disorders and Pelvic Organ Prolapse. https://medicine.yale.edu/obgyn/urogyn/UI-POP_patient_talk_23938_1095_5.pdf*

26. David Wise, Ph.D &Rodney Anderson, M.D. *A Headache in the Pelvis A New Understanding and Treatment for Prostatitis and Chronic Pelvic Pain Syndrome* (National Center For pelvic Pain Research, 2012), 90.

27. Ibid, 118.

28. Eric Franklin, *Pelvic Power: Mind/Body Exercises for Strength, Flexibility, Posture and Balance for Men and Women.* (Elysian Editions Princeton Book Company, 2002) 34.

29. Liz Koch, quoted in Danielle Prohom Olsen, "The Psoas: Muscle of the Soul," *The Body Divine*, https://bodydivineyoga.wordpress.com/2011/03/23/the-psoas-muscle-of-the-soul/

30. Danielle Olsen, *'Muscle of the Soul' Might Be Causing You Fear and Anxiety* http://expandedconsciousness.com/2016/04/08/muscle-of-the-soul-might-be-causing-you-fear-and-anxiety/

31. Donna Holleman, *Centering Down* (Tipograffia, Guistina, Firenze. 1981), 20.

32. Richard Schleip Ph.D, *New Perspectives in Fascia Research*. The International Fascia Research Congress. Washington, D.C. November, 2015, https://www.youtube.com/watch?v=iUj0XE0O6Fk

33. John Maxwell Taylor, in conversation with the author, 2016

34. Lipton, Bruce, *The Biology of Belief* (Hay House, 2008), xv.

35. Leigh Fortson, "Embrace, Release, Heal: An Empowering Guide to Talking About, Thinking About and Treating Cancer. Interview with Dr. Bruce Lipton" February 7, 2012. *http://www.embracehealingcancer.com/bios.html*

36. Bruce Lipton, M.D. Ph.D, *The Biology of Belief* (Hay House, 2005), xiii.

37. Bruce Lipton, M.D. Ph.D, *The Biology of Belief* (Hay House, 2005), 107.

38. Ibid, 59.

39. Ibid, 60.

40. Haley Cohen, "The Game of Clones," *Vanity Fair*, July 21, 2015 http://www.vanityfair.com/news/2015/07/polo-horse-cloning-adolfo-cambiaso

41. Bruce Lipton, M.D. Ph.D, *The Biology of Belief* (Hay House, 2005), 103.

42. Ibid, 58.

43. Ibid, 53-54.

44. Ibid, 55.

45. Ibid, 54.

46. ibid 55.

47. Phillip Beach, *Muscles and Meridians, The Manipulation of Shape* (Churchill Livingston Elsevier, 2010) page 1

48. Ibid, page 137

49. Bruce Lipton, M.D. Ph.D, *The Biology of Belief*. Hay House, 2005 page 113

50. Thomas Hübl, *Mystical Principles 2* (Thomas Hübl Online Course), 2015

51. Leigh Fortson, "Embrace, Release, Heal: An Empowering Guide to Talking About, Thinking About and Treating Cancer. Interview with Dr. Bruce Lipton," February 7, 2012. *http://www.embracehealingcancer.com/bios.html*

52. Eckhart Tolle, *The Power of Now: A Guide to Spiritual Enlightenment* (Vancouver, BC: Namaste Publishing, 2004), 111.

53. Lynne McTaggart, *The Intention Experiment, The Power of Conscious Intention, Part 1*, July, 2012. https://www.youtube.com/watch?v=dTHCusfKiZk

54. Albert Einstein, from the film *Atomic Physics* (1948), J. Arthur Rank Organization, Ltd.

55. Albert Einstein, quoted in Bruce Lipton, *Spontaneous Evolution* (Hay House, 2009), 269.

56. Brian Goodwin, *Nature's Due: Healing Our Fragmented Culture* (Floris Books, 2007), 177.

57. Robert Lanza, M.D. *Biocentrism: How Life and Consciousness are the Keys to Understanding the True Nature of the Universe* (BenBella Books, 2010), 2.

58. Ibid, 2.

59. Stephen Busby, Higher Consciousness Online Course, "Awakening to a Higher Frequency of Life," December 9, 2015

60. ibid, 160.

61. Belleruth Naparstek, *Invisible Heroes: Survivors of Trauma and How They Heal* (New York, NY: Bantam 2004)

62. Demetrovics, Z. Kurimay, T. Psychiatr Hung, "Exercise Addiction: A Literature Review," 2008; 23(2) 129-41. *Review Hungarian* PMID: 18956613

ABOUT THE AUTHOR

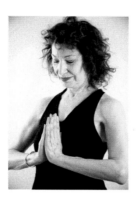

GINNY NADLER IS the founder and CEO of Core Body Wisdom®, which delivers the highest quality wellness initiatives and care to individuals, businesses, healthcare providers and organizations. The core of Ginny's approach is Structural ReAlignment Integration® (SRI) which draws on her years as a wellness educator and body alignment specialist to support individuals with stressed and in pain structures to be pain free and rediscover freedom in movement. Ginny studied yoga in the B.K.S. Iyengar Tradition for years before deciding to seek more creative ways to discover where imbalance and distortion arise in human structure and psyche with a focus on releasing trauma in the pelvic floor. She cofounded the first comprehensive wellness center on the East Coast and also created The Urban Global Healing Center where she participated in and helped develop a wellness program for young women incarcerated and offered a wide range of wellness education services. Ginny works with the worldwide Pocket Project Training with 150 others from 39 countries, exploring cultural agreements and global collective trauma (that live within us all). She also consults with individuals to help awaken them to the trauma that exists in their cell structures and collaborates with practitioners of other modalities seeking a deeper framework for their own approach to movement, trauma, and pain management.

www.corebodywisdom.com

Made in the USA
Monee, IL
27 July 2024

62757766R00159